RADICAL RESILIENCE

K. Sparrow, MD

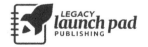

LEGACY launch pad PUBLISHING

Contents

This book is dedicated to scientific researchers across the globe whose curiosity and dogged work on problems large and small lead to countless incremental discoveries setting the stage for unexpected, extraordinary quantum leaps in knowledge. As in nature, transformation can happen gradually, and then, seemingly all at once.

Preface

"A crisis is an opportunity riding a dangerous wind."
—*Chinese proverb*

For most of my life, I traveled a traditional medical career path. Born and raised in the San Francisco Bay Area, I graduated in Biochemistry from UC Berkeley. I worked in the lab of a famous biochemist, Dr. Daniel D. Koshland Jr, before enrolling in medical school. I had seriously considered a research career but I didn't think I had the chops. I also felt that I would have more options by getting a medical degree. After completing my MD degree at Tulane University, my residency training followed in pediatrics at the University of California, Los Angeles (UCLA) and anesthesiology at the University of California, Irvine (UCI). These residencies led to a long-term position as an anesthesiologist in San Francisco. But shortly after moving there, I started having allergy symptoms.

I was no stranger to allergies, having suffered from hay fever growing up, but I thought I had outgrown them. Even so, by the end of the workday, I would sometimes feel my chest tightening with some wheezing, or an attack of severe allergic rhinitis—sniffling, sneezing, itchy red eyes, the works. It would be particularly bad when I was on call at night, with more pronounced wheezing. I had various rashes, especially on my face and hands. And I learned quickly to never touch my eyes with or without gloves.

Since I was familiar with allergies from my childhood and intermittently since then, I made light of the symptoms and other than using eye drops occasionally, I learned to live with them. I had some skin testing, but nothing too significant surfaced. After nearly 10 years of allergy affliction, a blood assay was finally developed to detect an allergy to latex. At the time, latex was found in all surgical gloves, and I couldn't simply wear some alternative. Latex gloves contained powder, and that powder saturated with latex was in the air in all operating rooms, delivery suites, emergency rooms, intensive care units and recovery rooms. Latex was everywhere my duties as an anesthesiologist took me.

The chief allergist at my hospital insisted that I step away from my position. Latex allergies could be very severe, sometimes so much so that they could even be triggered by the smell of car tires. In the worst cases, patients' pulmonary issues could get bad enough to be disabling. In short, my latex allergy was serious and it was not going away. This life-shattering news was softened by the fact that the hospital administration assured me that latex gloves would be discontinued within a year or so. With that in mind, I took a leave of absence, planning to return once they had been phased out.

I decided to treat this unwanted and unexpected break in my career as a rare opportunity to have an adventure with my young family. Since my husband was a real estate entrepreneur and could live anywhere, we decided to move to Barcelona for a year with our three young children.

Within three weeks of moving to Barcelona, I began looking for a way to expand my career opportunities in addition to learning Spanish. I considered taking acupuncture training since it had been on my radar before I left the United States. Pain management is a branch of anesthesiology, and since acupuncture could ease patients' pain, it seemed like a good fit for me. I figured it might be possible to add acupuncture to my skill set before returning to my position in San Francisco—and being involved in a school setting would also help immerse me in the local language and culture.

A Professional Crisis of Commitment: What Am I Doing?

The first set of lectures captured my attention. As far back as 2600 BC, the ancients recognized the association between lung health and skin afflictions, as was the case with my own allergies. They also tied kidney and ear function together as well, which my training as a pediatrician supported—I'd been taught to look for kidney abnormalities if a newborn's ear was deformed. Because of connections like these, I tried to keep an open mind to this new system of constructs, though I will admit I was a skeptic.

I was resistant at the beginning of my acupuncture training to much of the material I was learning—extremely resistant, if I can be frank. I balked completely, however, when we had our first hands-on lesson. We were learning a procedure that involved piercing the patient's back with a tiny scalpel nick, applying a suction cup and draining blood. It was the ancient procedure of "cupping," made more alarming by adding a type of bloodletting. I was familiar with cupping from being a pediatric resident at UCLA; Hispanic families would sometimes bring in their children with bruised-red circular marks on their backs, and we doctors would all shake our heads, aghast at what we considered a superstition. *What in the world have I gotten myself into?* I thought. *Why am I wasting my time with this utter nonsense?* I'm sad to say I also wondered what all of my medical colleagues, not to mention my biochemistry research pals, would think of me if I kept studying acupuncture.

Despite my reservations, I stuck with my training. I also started getting twice-weekly acupuncture treatments at the school I was attending to help manage my allergies and experience acupuncture firsthand. I was extremely curious how the treatments would feel and if they could help me as my classes and teachers indicated they would. In the middle of this course of treatments, I was reading to my oldest daughter in her bedroom one night when out of nowhere, it felt like I had been heavily dusted with some kind of diabolical itching powder. As I sneezed over and over and over again, my daughter looked at me alarmed and asked me what was going on. I told her that I'd be fine but that we'd have to finish the reading another time. The fit progressed to irritated, itchy eyes and a swollen, bloated face. My throat went from scratchy to swollen and I started to drool uncontrollably. It was a full-blown allergy attack, the worst I had ever had.

As a doctor, I knew there was a chance that my condition could deteriorate rapidly; the attack I was having could lead to my throat closing entirely, and I didn't want my kids to be the ones to have call the Barcelona equivalent of 911. Because of that, I started preparing to go to the emergency room. I called my husband, who was out with friends, and told him he should come home immediately—and though he was initially grumpy his night was cut short, he saw the sorry state I was in and understood how serious the situation was. I knew what awaited me in the emergency room would be an intravenous line, treatment with steroids, epinephrine injections and anti-histamines—but even though all of that would've treated my symptoms, considering all those medical interventions made me pause.

I was battling with my logical inner voice: *Use your medical training for your own good, for heaven's sake, and go to the hospital where you belong—in more ways than one!* But the curious scientist in me was performing an experiment. I was trying an alternative treatment for allergies through acupuncture, and I deeply wanted to complete the experiment, not taint its results with a medical bailout. My scientist's voice insisted against jumping to Western solutions, as contrarian as that sounds, and eventually won out.

Instead of going to the hospital, I took a long, thorough shower and my condition improved somewhat. Though I still had hay fever type-symptoms, the acute swelling sensation in my throat had subsided. I went to sleep, satisfied that I'd avoided the hospital's modern medical interventions and preserved the integrity of my experiment.

Crisis of Cure

The next day, I had an acupuncture treatment scheduled. With my eyes nearly swollen shut, I went to see my Chinese acupuncture teacher who'd been treating my allergies for weeks. I arrived wearing big dark glasses to cover my red, swollen eyes so I wouldn't alarm other students or people on the bus. After I explained to him what had happened, to my utter and absolute astonishment, he was not a bit concerned. After one look at my ravaged face and eyes, he gently replaced my dark sunglasses. "You'll be fine now," he said. "You've finally expelled the perversive energy."

My teacher, an old-school Chinese practitioner who hailed from Shanghai, was right. At first, I didn't believe him, but as the months went on and I was free of hay fever, rashes and other symptoms that had been with me for years, it dawned on me that something really *had* shifted. In Western medicine, the diagnosis of such severe allergies dictated that I would need to take inhalers, nasal sprays and antihistamines for life to combat my allergies. My teacher, on the other hand, was confident that my body could control them—and it did. Though I've occasionally had mild reactions since that unforgettable night so many years ago, my allergies have basically disappeared.

A Crisis of Curiosity and New Beginnings

My allergy attack and subsequent reduction in symptoms is what in acupuncture circles is called a "crisis of cure." It means that a patient's symptoms can get worse before they disappear. Though many people have experienced a crisis of cure, the phenomenon is difficult to define scientifically. Given my background, I struggled to believe it was real since I couldn't explain it—even though it had happened to me. I'd experienced a dramatic life event that had turned my thinking upside down, but it had also created an opportunity for a new beginning. In my case, my remarkable "crisis of cure" made me start taking my acupuncture training seriously.

I now see that night of the severe allergic reaction as an initiation—a breakthrough into seeing health, medicine, longevity and science in a new way. It forced me to abandon the "givens" in my thinking, though I stayed true to my fondness for science. I started looking for a deeper understanding of my experience. I wanted to explain scientifically and physiologically what had happened to me instead of writing it off as chance, placebo or wishful thinking. To that end, I became acquainted with many different, rapidly evolving fields and concepts in medicine, such as immunology, autonomic dysfunction, stress, complexity science and systems biology. Now that I have put many years into that process, I have become an unwitting and very minor participant in the fascinating trajectory of acupuncture's role in medicine.

Acupuncture has evolved from being a fringe novelty to an increasingly accepted therapy that can be studied in animals and humans. Some acupuncture research has helped inform other branches of medicine by helping show how the body reacts to injury. It has provided new insights into pain management, brain reactivity and other phenomena involved in how healing, well-being and resilience can occur.

Learning to Seek

I never did return to my anesthesia position. It took years to eliminate all latex from hospitals. By that time, I had established my own acupuncture practice and never looked back.

My own research into acupuncture has not been an academic pursuit per se. In trying to make sense of my experience, I developed a keen interest in scientific acupuncture research. A large part of my obsession with current research has also been pragmatic. It helps me get better results for my patients, because most medicine, acupuncture included, is not like the law of gravity. Acupuncture doesn't always work, and as a practitioner, that motivates you to keep learning—because you want it to always work! You want it to be like gravity!

As an anesthesiologist, I come from a field of medicine where practitioners can virtually *always* get a patient to become unconscious. It can sometimes take more drugs and some finesse and there may be side effects, but most of the time, it is almost as reliable as gravity. But in many parts of medicine things don't always work that way. It is more complicated than that, as we will see in the upcoming chapters.

Patients often say to me that they "believe" in acupuncture. I remind them that acupuncture works on lab animals, so belief is not necessary (though keeping their appointments is). By following and using the science, I can't help but think that acupuncture will become more effective, more consistent and more "believable." In a way, it may become a bit more like gravity.

Why This Book Now?

All the threads of science and research that I have gathered and posted on my website and blog, the observational studies I've performed and presented at Acupuncture and Neuromodulation conferences, were a record of my exploration but not arranged in any useful way. Originally, I wanted to organize the material just for myself, but the more I read, the more I realized that patients, physicians, lay acupuncturists and the public didn't realize how much science there was behind Chinese medicine's philosophy and application. And this very science also helps explain other related treatments and even some currently popular "health hacks."

All of the above are major reasons for writing this book, though if I'm fully honest with myself, I might also still be justifying myself to all the dismissive voices of medical and biochemical research colleagues I can hear in my head. Perhaps because of the profound skepticism I once harbored, and which continued as I searched for the scientific basis for acupuncture's results, I feel well-positioned to share what I've learned. Scientific inquiry has doubt and skepticism as constant companions, and both have plagued me throughout my process of tracking down and blogging about acupuncture medical studies. But they have also led me to more robust and reliable conclusions. We all need to question studies and their results and not accept subpar studies that match our own biases.

Seeking to Learn

There is a Buddhist concept that says a full cup can accept no more water. Likewise, a mind full of what we think we know can receive no knowledge. As readers, to truly accept some of the concepts I'm about to share here require opening your mind to new ways of thinking and to some alternative para-

Preface

digms and mental models. I hope you will let your curiosity lead you while we tour the fascinating and elegant systems of the body and bridge the secrets of ancient practice with cutting-edge science.

We will begin with a bit of the wisdom of ancient practitioners contained in the parable of Dr. One.

Chapter 1
In Search of Doctor One: Embracing Nature's Laws for Radical Prevention and Long Life

"Without sensitive regard to the larger scheme of the universal law, modern science and technology will continue to produce disturbance and even destruction to all life on earth. In the modern age, the East can indeed offer the West a philosophy of balance and harmony that is not only urgently needed but necessary for the survival of human civilization."
—Maoshing Ni, *The Yellow Emperor's Classic of Medicine*

In the bygone world where ancient Chinese practice was the mainstream of the day, medical practitioners taught that fostering and maintaining deep energetic balance in body and mind would lead to robust resilience and resistance to disease and harm. This balance would not only lead to more energy and better mood but would also allow for enviable longevity of 100 years and beyond. They believed that generating a tough constitution would provide profound prevention, allowing patients to withstand toxins, trauma and illness. This idea of radical prevention was not based on testing for illness or getting vaccinated, which makes up much of our concept of prevention today, but deep inner stability. And it was the ultimate treatment goal.

This potential for the deep balance that leads to robust health described by the ancient practitioners sounds alluring, but it also seems exotic or even preposterous today. Our modern lives feel so far removed from day-to-day life in 2600 BC China. Our environments are rife with pollutants and dangers. We are chronically stressed out while the threat of cancer, heart disease and dementia loom in our thinking.

But what if we *could* stay healthy, stave off illness and—most seductive of all—live longer? What if we could make the body stronger and sturdier to ward off problems before they take hold, as ancient practice teaches? Wouldn't that represent a truly elegant solution? Yes, there is more than a bit of a utopian vision in this, but parts of this vision are not as outlandish or unrealistic as they might sound. And that ideal is what we will be exploring in this book.

Ancient Chinese philosophy encouraged a harmonious, balanced lifestyle, and Chinese medicine was an inherent part of that. It comprised a complex collection of observations, constructs and treatments. Many aspects of this knowledge base have not withstood the test of time, but others have. Some tried-and-true ancient teachings have the potential to lead the way to new avenues of treatment and research, as well as provide practical and safe ways to optimize health, leading to a longer and more vital life. In modern medicine, longevity science is quite new, but not so in the teachings of Chinese medicine, where longevity was an intrinsic goal. There, the concept of fostering a sturdy sense of resilience that led to a longer life is interwoven into the fabric of ancient teachings and dictums.

To understand this, our journey begins with a few of these basic tenets of Chinese medicine, found in the parable of The Three Doctors.

The Ancient Legend of the Three Doctors

A story from ancient Chinese medicine teaches that the best, most sought-after doctor, Dr. One, kept patients well and cured them if they became ill or injured. He achieved this through basic interventions, such as acupuncture, massage, moxibustion, herbal treatments, lifestyle recommendations and avoiding harm. Patients flocked to him, and his waiting room was overflowing. Dr. One's patients were more than willing to take the time and effort to see him, because they could see that they were less likely to get sick by coming to him. They could feel better and sleep well. By checking on patients periodically, assessing them with the tools of the day (pulse and tongue diagnosis and skin tone, to name a few) and offering treatment, Dr. One could give his patients a better chance of avoiding harm. Dr. One could also cure patients if they did become sick or injured, but that was not why he was famous. People would visit him in health as well as sickness to keep themselves optimized.

The second-best doctor, Dr. Two, could cure patients once they got sick, but he had little to offer in between illnesses. The worst doctor, Dr. Three, made patients worse with his care and was called a butcher behind his back. When I learned this parable during my acupuncture training, I filed it away as a quirky bit of Chinese lore. But I never forgot about those three doctors.

I will use comparisons between the respective approaches and abilities of these doctors throughout this book to illustrate key points, but first, let's consider a little about the current state of public health and the medical system in the West.

Is America's Medical System the Best in the World?

Every day, we're confronted with a mind-numbing variety of debilitating and life-threatening diseases. Our family and friends have fallen victim to the leading causes of death in the USA—heart disease, cancer, stroke, chronic lower respiratory disease (chronic bronchitis, emphysema and asthma), Alzheimer's and diabetes. More recently, the COVID-19 virus has taken a deadly toll in what we hope was a once-in-a-century pandemic.

According to the Centers for Medicare & Medicaid Services, as a nation, we spend over four trillion dollars or $12,914 per person annually on healthcare.[1] And yet, by some estimates, that same healthcare is one of the top causes of injury and death. Research at Johns Hopkins and Arizona State University concludes that between 250,000 and 400,000 deaths yearly are due to medical error.[2] We routinely state that America has the best medical services in the world, but do we? The grim fact is that among wealthy nations, we spend more and yet still come in last on basic health and healthcare delivery metrics. Infant mortality statistics paint a bleak picture of the US, too; we rank worse than Russia, Cuba, Uruguay and Poland and have rates almost three times higher than Norway's.[3] So, is there a better way?

To a degree, we all are creatures of habit; our expectations are set by what we have done before and how we have thought and been taught. With this in mind, my goal is to bend and even substitute some of our current conventional wisdom and mental models around health and medical care. For example, it is commonplace in our society to favor and believe in the dramatic, the expensive and the white-coated solution as we dismiss the unglamorous but important work of public health mainstays. Conversely, in the realm of acupuncture, I've seen patients confronted by healing episodes that defy what they understand. But instead of accepting or trying to understand their positive results, they argue with them, discount them and dismiss them as placebo or chance—though if they'd received the same results through surgery, they would likely accept them as a cure wholeheartedly.

4

I make this comparison not to be critical of patients, but to illustrate a simple but foundational point I will return to again and again in this book: our mental models have a dramatic influence on us, and they can shape our behavior to an astonishing degree.

Translating Ancient Teachings into Modern Science

The world of Dr. One is a place that defies some of our closely held understanding of how healing works. It challenges the "fix it" aspect of modern medicine's implicit, powerful metaphor of *man-as-machine*. According to this mental model, a person's body is a machine that needs to be "fixed" through drastic interventions. In some severe cases, this model can be accurate and valuable, producing medical miracles that no one would want to abandon. But Dr. One teaches that with smaller and more careful interventions by staying well and balanced, we can sometimes better avoid the dangers surrounding us, and live longer. This is a radical proposition in the context of how we view health and illness in the 21st century, and anything "radical" can make us feel uneasy and take some getting used to.

By probing the scientific underpinnings of Dr. One's methods, we will hopefully stretch our mental models and become more comfortable with Dr. One's sustained, proactive approach. Three principles will help us bridge the explanatory gap between these ancient teachings and modern science:

1. Balance
2. Hormesis
3. Systems Synergy, or "It All Spins Together"

Balance: The Art of Maintaining Homeostasis

Balance is a key concept in Ancient Chinese medicine. To better understand the importance of balance, consider a washing machine. A washing machine must be balanced to operate efficiently and avoid rocking wildly out of control, and the same is true of the way our bodies work. The principle of balance is alive and well in the modern concept of *homeostasis*, the process by which a biological system maintains equilibrium through many regulatory mechanisms. Another simple analogy is your furnace's thermostat as a regulatory or feedback mechanism. In the body, multiple sophisticated feedback loops ensure that the body regulates everything from temperature to heart rate to immune function. These feedback loops correct minor disturbances and keep the body operating smoothly without spiraling out of control like an unbalanced washing machine.

Dr. One knows this secret. He does his best to "do no harm" and uses time-honored techniques to keep the body balanced while advising on avoiding damaging habits and reducing stress. But to keep our systems resistant, tough and ready to respond to toxins, illness and heartbreak, it must encounter small challenges through a process known as *hormesis*.

Hormesis: The Small Challenges That Can Lead to Big Results

The term hormesis comes from the ancient Greek *hormáein*, meaning "to set in motion, impel, urge on." Hormesis introduces low-grade challenges to the body, which stress it without causing damage, such as exercise, stretching and calorie restriction. Acupuncture also qualifies as a hormetic challenge.

You might intuitively think that completely avoiding

mental and physical stressors would lead to a safe, long and healthy life. But not so. We don't want to become hothouse flowers that cannot withstand the challenges of the natural environment. The body needs challenges and nudging to stay tough, prevent illness and enjoy optimum health. The current fields of immunology and longevity science give us insight into the powerful workings of the subtle and not-so-subtle feedback systems that maintain homeostasis or balance. These systems help keep us resilient in the face of life's challenges and allow us to see how small challenges can prod these systems to our advantage.

This relates to the intrinsic teaching in Chinese medicine that all systems affect each other. It is the basis of the perhaps-overused phrase "a holistic approach," though the core concept is still powerfully important.

Systems Synergy, or "It All Spins Together"

From deep in our evolutionary DNA, we have learned to distrust the unfamiliar. For instance, our immune system rejects foreign matter, and, at an emotional level, we might reject foreigners or new ideas as dangerous. Thomas Kuhn, the towering philosopher of science, said it best: before a new scientific idea or paradigm can be fully accepted, the old generation must die off so a new generation of scientists, not set in their ways, can accept and build on that idea.

According to ancient teachings, there is a circular system of generation between organ systems, as "it all spins together." If one organ is depleted, it will affect the entire generative cycle of all organs. And conversely, as taught in Chinese medicine, when you become more robust and balanced in one area, you become stronger in others too. When you treat one symptom or sign of imbalance, it can stabilize the entire body. And because our bodies' systems are a web of many feedback loops, the changes can be gradual or seem to happen all at once.

"It all spins together" requires reframing some of our thinking about health and well-being. This reframing, in turn, requires having an open mind and being willing to "unlearn" some of what we think we know to allow ourselves a glimpse of what may be possible. In the biography *Steve Jobs,* author Walter Isaacson wrote that Jobs understood the necessity of a deep belief that big goals *could be done* as a prerequisite to actually doing them.[4] The same is true of embracing an effective new approach to medicine.

It begins with considering: What if the ancient practitioners were right? The ancients believed (and saw with their own eyes) that there were steps you could take to achieve a long and healthy life. In short, *they believed it could be done.* Once we do the same, the next challenge is to find new strategies of thinking that can help us remember to think in systems instead of parts—to think outside of dogma and more in line with nature as the ancients did.

Biomimicry: Learning from Nature

At a book fair, I heard biomimicry entrepreneur Jay Harman, author of *The Shark's Paintbrush: Biomimicry and How Nature Is Inspiring Innovation,* explain how he had developed a small turbine mixer six inches high by four inches wide that was capable of mixing a 40-foot deep reservoir of stagnant water as large as a football field—using only the power of three lightbulbs.[5] Using his small mixer, clean tap water could be produced from this reservoir using 80 percent less disinfectant and 90 percent less energy. So, what was so special about his rotor? How did he do this? The answer comes from a relatively new field of scientific research called biomimicry.

From Harman's years of field research, he knew that nature always used the least energy and materials to get a job done. As one reviewer of Harman's book explained, "Nature [has] 3.8 billion years of design experience...and can teach profound lessons on how things should be made and how they work."

As Harman observed, nature finds the most energy-efficient ways to move fluids, and it is never in a straight line. Instead, fluids move in spirals, like the whirlpool in the drain of your kitchen sink, which is more efficient. As Harman estimates in his book, two-thirds of the energy we spend pulling fluids out of the ground is wasted by forcing fluids to move in straight lines instead of using spiral flow geometry found in nature, as spiral flow geometry takes advantage of turbulence instead of wasting energy by fighting it.

With these insights, Harman was determined to optimize the design of his turbine by mimicking the shapes of natural spiral flows, but soon found that the 3D geometry of whirlpools was very challenging to reproduce. Though Harman had no modern tools available to create a whirlpool and perfectly capture its shape, he ingeniously solved this problem by freezing a whirlpool and then developing his single-blade rotor and all its astonishing capabilities from the ice model.

Harman sees biomimicry as inspiration for better design and a way to help Mother Nature survive by decreasing our energy consumption. Similarly, practitioners can potentially find more effective and less harmful treatment methods by applying some of the same principles: understanding that the human body is a complex and interconnected natural system, not a bunch of separate "parts."

The parallel here is that by backing away from the *man-as-machine* model and a reductionist mindset, and by focusing instead on harnessing or incorporating the natural feedback systems our bodies have evolved over millennia, we can get better, safer results. One of the most powerful systems we can focus on is our autonomic nervous system, which controls our body's stress response. A whole range of our bodily functions —from gut health to immunity, pain and mood—are profoundly sensitive to our autonomic balance.

The Power of Autonomic Balance for Well-Being and Long Life

Autonomic balance refers to the coordination between the two branches of the autonomic nervous system: the sympathetic nervous system and the parasympathetic nervous system. The autonomic nervous system plays a vital role in regulating various bodily functions, including heart rate, blood pressure, respiration, digestion and stress response. This yin/yang system balances fight-or-flight and rest-and-digest aspects of our unconscious physiology and represents a crucial response to physical and mental challenges.

Inflammation is tightly correlated with autonomic imbalance and is increasingly being found to be a feature of most modern diseases. We now know that inflammation, which is susceptible to the autonomic nervous system, is a pivotal factor in cardiac disease and cancer.[6] Both of these diseases are huge destabilizers of the body's balance and leading causes of death—and though we don't often think of it in these terms, death is always the ultimate result of the body's systems spiraling out of control. Because inflammation can be "silent," preventing it by balancing the autonomic nervous system through exercise, meditation and acupuncture can be a helpful and effective treatment strategy. By doing so, you can improve your autonomic balance, thereby improving mood, calming anxiety and boosting immunity, all leading to less overall inflammation and better sleep and digestion.

Using small stressors, such as the stimulation of acupuncture needles in one area, can affect our overall autonomic balance, leading to positive and outsized "global" results on our well-being and longevity. As we achieve autonomic balance, we allow and coax our systems to spin or spiral together for better health and longer life, a little like Harman's small but mighty turbine that can spin an entire reservoir of water by harnessing nature's principles.

Modern Evidence for Ancient Practice and Making the Invisible Visible

For centuries, ancient Chinese medicine practitioners have demonstrated remarkable improvements in the health of their patients. Now, advances in modern science, computing capabilities and the emerging fields of systems biology (how physiological systems affect each other) and complexity science (a mathematical way of measuring complex systems) can demonstrate subtle physiological changes and validate these ancient concepts. Many can be quantified; they are not abstract and do not need to be taken on faith. When it comes to ancient lore, the invisible has become visible, and modern science has evidence to back it up.

Our guiding hope in this is, yes, to live long, but above all, to live *well*—to "live deep and suck out all the marrow of life" as Thoreau said.[7] And yes, this is a moonshot, but keeping that vision in mind as our ultimate destination makes the journey more compelling and worth taking. We are trying to achieve radical resilience—a sort of radical prevention that keeps us flourishing so we have a better chance of being healthy and living longer.

As we discuss Dr. One's approach in the coming chapters, we will focus on the science so that the concepts may become less foreign and more convincing. Doing so will mean embracing new mental models, avoiding perverse incentives in our medical system and being open to a new sense of *what might be possible*. By introducing these ancient principles through the eyes of modern science, I hope that these ideas will become familiar, feasible, and above all, useful to you.

Though there is still an enormous and vital role for an army of Dr. Twos, there is a desperate need for Dr. Ones. By combining ancient practices with modern strategies, there is potential for radical prevention and increased longevity by developing deep resilience of body and mind.

Chapter 2
Do No Harm

"It takes a wise doctor to know when not to prescribe."
–Baltasar Gracián, *The Art of Worldly Wisdom*, 1647

Micah's Story

Former baseball pitcher Micah Bowie was in excruciating pain. After years of playing in the major and minor leagues, he lay curled in bed, sobbing. "My wife had a husband who was degrading, going from fighting through anything as an athlete to lying in bed crying in a ball all day long. It was horrible for her and my kids to watch," Bowie told the *San Francisco Chronicle*.[1]

Bowie's frequent back pain, which was caused by tears associated with his L4-5 and L5-S1 (fourth and fifth lumbar, fifth lumbar first sacral) vertebrae, intensified after he retired in 2008. Bowie and his wife Keeley investigated surgery or stem-cell treatment as he became more incapacitated and his treatments less effective. Initially, doctors recommended a double-disk fusion procedure with a warning that he would probably face repeat surgeries for the rest of his life. Then doctors suggested a spinal-cord stimulator, an internal device that blocks nerve pain signals. After a successful week-long trial in August 2016, he had the device implanted.

No more than a month later, Bowie awoke in unspeakable pain, struggling to breathe. It was the beginning of innumerable ambulance trips, hospital stays and consultations with various back experts. "The worst part was that no one believed me. It was a nightmare scenario," Bowie told the *Chronicle*.[2]

Experts were mystified until X-rays revealed that the device's battery had migrated from a subcutaneous pocket and ripped through his liver, diaphragm and right lung. Doctors removed parts of Bowie's lungs and repaired his diaphragm, but his condition continued to worsen. The oxygen levels in his blood dropped. His neurological function deteriorated. His liver, heart, kidneys and adrenal glands were all damaged. Even though doctors moved the battery to Bowie's hip, they wouldn't consider it the cause of his breathing issues.

Major League Baseball arranged a consultation with a thoracic surgeon at an internationally renowned clinic who discovered Bowie's lungs had electrical burns.

"You're being shocked to death," he was told. He was also told his situation was untreatable and that he should get his affairs in order, which was polite speak for "Go home and die." Fortunately, a St. Louis surgeon who'd repaired Bowie's groin injury in 2007 finally stepped in and asked him to visit. Bowie was admitted to the hospital and the surgeon removed his spinal cord stimulator after many other doctors had refused to touch it. "They stopped it from electrically killing me," said Bowie, who was left with just eight percent of his lung capacity.

How did Bowie get into this miserable state of affairs? This chapter is about the powerful calculation of risk versus benefit, and how the consequences of that calculation can be substantial in medicine. You'll discover why sometimes the best course of action is to do nothing, and yet doing nothing can be one of the most difficult courses to take. Along the way, we'll see that Charlie Munger and UCSF professor Rita Redberg, both experts in vastly different fields, see the wisdom in the maxim that less can be more. And consider how even the inspirational Cures Act, an act of congress to fund cancer research, may be favoring the wrong priorities. And with the mental models in mind that helped to seal Bowie's fate, we will carefully consider his case.

Three Strikes against Micah Bowie

Bowie's is a heartbreaking and maddening case, and it encapsulates the importance of the Hippocratic Oath: "First, do no harm," or as philosopher Gracián says, "It takes a wise doctor to know when not to prescribe."[3] Remembering the fable of the good reputation of Dr. One and the bad reputation of Dr. Three, we will discover that "doing no harm" is not as straightforward as it might seem. Sometimes, it can be devilishly difficult. I make no specific judgment about the doctors who treated Bowie or the treatment he received. Undoubtedly, the doctors who cared for him were doing their best in a challenging situation. Instead, my goal is to look at the mental models and "common wisdom" that were working against them.

Bowie was a high-profile professional baseball player with excruciating back pain, and in all likelihood, according to the *Chronicle* article, he faced a lifetime of surgeries. The X-rays he received probably revealed a serious problem, and spinal cord stimulation was considered a less invasive approach than repeated surgeries. Fair enough. But in his story, I see signals of entrenched and prevailing counterforces that could've tilted his healthcare specialists into dangerous Dr. Three territory.

Bowie had three strikes against him:

Strike One: Bowie was a person of prominence, which put added pressure on the doctors. The reputational impact of treating him could've easily tipped many decisions from *doing nothing* to *doing something*.

Strike Two: Bowie was in great pain, suffering so much that it conferred extra urgency upon the doctors to find some treatment that would provide him with relief.

Strike Three: Bowie lived near a major metropolitan area with many "smart" doctors, "cool medical toys" and sophisticated treatment options.

But wait, you might be thinking, *how are these are all strikes against him?* I will explain—but first, let's explore why doctors often pursue treatment even though *less can be more.*

Wisdom Is Prevention: Avoiding the Bad

Charlie Munger, the business partner of Warren Buffett and vice chairman of Berkshire Hathaway, is famous for a presumably tongue-in-cheek quote: "All I want to know is where I'm going to die, so I'll never go there."[4] What he was getting at is that avoiding the bad is often more powerful than seeking the good. He lives by a pithy saying that Dr. One would likely agree with: "Wisdom is Prevention." In business decision-making, avoiding stupidity is the more effective road to follow rather than seeking brilliance. The parallel in medicine is that avoiding harm can be more effective than seeking a dazzling solution.

The incidence of problems caused by medical errors is staggering and, according to Johns Hopkins research, the third leading cause of death in the US.[5] To stay firmly in the realm of Dr. One and steer clear of Dr. Three, we need to know when to avoid rather than treat. Most people, of course, expect doctors to treat them—to *do something*—and they believe in the virtues of modern medicine. Typically, Americans credit about 80 percent of the increase in life expectancy since the mid-1800s to modern medicine, as revealed in a Brigham Young University study.[6] It is a common attitude we hear when people say things like, "It's wonderful what doctors can do today." But the Brigham Young University researchers also wrote: "The public grossly overestimates how much of our increased lifespan should be attributed to medical care and is largely unaware of the critical role played by public health and improved social conditions determinants."

As the researchers explain, life expectancy has dramatically improved primarily because of improvements in basic sanitation and decreased poverty, but the perception that medical care deserves the credit hinders funding for public health. And as they wrote, it "may also contribute to over-funding the medical sector of the economy and impede efforts to contain health care costs."

Robbing Prevention to Pay for Cures

Fighting Heart Disease: Move, Lose and Clean Up Your Act

We can take charge of our personal well-being in many ways without costly medical interventions. Consider heart disease, the most common killer in the US, responsible for one in every five deaths.[7] It's reasonable to believe that medication and surgery would make a huge difference, but these approaches are nothing compared to simple, moderate lifestyle changes. In a meta-study that pooled data from tens of thousands of people over a 21-year period, one study from Massachusetts General Hospital researchers found that people deemed at high familial risk of heart disease cut their risk in half if they satisfied three of four criteria:

1. Didn't smoke (even if they smoked in the past).
2. Were not obese (although they could be overweight).
3. Exercised once a week.
4. Ate more real food and less processed food. [8]

But consider the $6.3 billion 21st Century Cures Act, a law created in part to bolster cancer research, and which passed through Congress to widespread acclaim. After all, who could argue with bolstering cancer research? Among others, the heads of the American Academy of Family Physicians and the American Public Health Association, as it turns out. Both argued against the law because it took $3.5 billion *away* from public-health efforts to instead fund research on medical technology and drugs, including the "cancer moonshot" first promoted by President Biden when he was vice president.[9]

The law took money away from programs like vaccination and smoking cessation that are known to *prevent* disease, and moved it to research and programs that might, eventually, *treat* disease. The act also allowed the FDA to approve new uses for drugs based on observational studies or anecdotal data. As a result of this law, pharmaceutical companies no longer have to give the FDA raw data, but rather their own "summary level" review of a drug's merits. This means that new drugs or procedures do not require rigorous peer review, a minimum requirement that is absolutely *essential* to ensure that a therapy actually works and provides more benefit than harm.

As we will discuss, this lack of rigor can be dangerous in many ways. Once these slapdash studies are given credence, there is no money to repeat them; they are simply accepted. Rita Redberg, a University of California, San Francisco (UCSF) cardiologist and editor of the Journal of the American Medical Association (JAMA Internal Medicine) wrote a series of articles called "Less is More."[10] In those articles, Dr. Redberg said, "Right now, people think that if a little health-care is good, then more healthcare is better, which is not always the case."

I attended a lecture where Dr. Redberg addressed the problem of drugs being released recklessly to patients. She referred to it as: "Once the train has left the station, you can't get it back syndrome."

I have found it is especially hard for people to question the idea that more medical treatments must inevitably lead to better outcomes. This deeply entrenched idea is a misconception that has multiple manifestations.

Dying to Treat: The Bias Towards Action over Risk versus Benefit Analysis

There's a bias towards action that Charlie Munger calls the "do something syndrome." Similarly, author and thinker Nassim Nicholas Talib coined the term *interventionistas* for people who come armed with solutions to problems without considering the long-term effects. Such individual health providers often deny that natural homeostatic mechanisms are sufficient and insist that *something needs to be done*. Yet often, the best course of action is minimal, just as Hippocrates reminds us. Talib also admonishes us to recognize that some systems self-correct; this is the very essence of homeostasis. In other words: *Doing nothing can get results.*

A simple rule for the health professional decision-maker is that intervention needs to prove its benefits, and those bene-fits need to be orders of magnitude greater than the non-inter-ventionist path. This reframes the crucial calculation of risk versus benefit that doctors face daily. We should unquestion-ably act when the benefits become orders of magnitude greater than doing nothing. Victims of car crashes and other accidents, patients with life-threatening cancer or people rushed to the hospital with a ruptured appendix all require immediate and decisive first-order action. But many of the most common ailments require prudence and thought. It can be counterproductive to be pressured to treat.

It goes against instinct not to treat, but when doctors fail to consider the second and third-order ramifications of their actions, they can make things worse and slip into the realm of Dr. Three. In modern medicine, there are some additional aspects of the industry that get in the way of the "less is more" ideal that physicians tend to embrace enthusiastically and all-too-easily. One of these is a phenomenon that I call "cool toys."

The Problem with "Cool Toys"

Advanced medical devices, or "cool toys," are a pernicious problem. From the doctor's standpoint, why perform regular surgery when you can use the latest, most technologically advanced robot? Why use old-fashioned verbal quizzes and flashcard drills to train anesthesiology residents when you can use a *cool* (exorbitantly expensive) state-of-the-art simulator? From the patient's standpoint, why not go for the latest procedure using the latest device? Isn't it bound to be the best? The answer is not at all.

It reminds me of a joke I first heard in med school: half the world needs vitamins, and the other half takes them. You could say the same for treatments and procedures. Over half the world needs more medical care, but the other half gets it —and too much of it. Like fancy expensive weapon systems that always, somehow, get deployed whether they are overkill or not, the most sophisticated medical devices seek a use. Medical interventions can also become "overkill." In fact, patients should want *other* people to be the clinical trial guinea pigs or early adopters of new drugs, surgeries or procedures.

The rule of thumb is to wait seven years after the release of a new treatment before accepting that it is safe and effective.

Spine stimulators, like the one Bowie received, are sophisticated, modern and use high-end implantable batteries. These expensive batteries require a trip to the radiology suite to place and replace them under fluoroscopy (a real-time X-ray that guides the surgeon in placement). The purpose of spine stimulators is to hijack the pain fibers and occupy them with a benign stimulation—a concept called "gating"—so that the pain is no longer perceived. Sometimes this works, and sometimes it does not.

Unfortunately for Bowie, the cutting-edge battery that ran his stimulator migrated into his lung. Because it was such a new device, the doctors had no idea how to deal with this turn of events. The result was a prolonged burning of Bowie's lungs and his body's systems spiraling out of control, with the potential result of death. While some surgeons might find it irresistible to play with the latest cool toys, there's also another related widespread preference for groundbreaking "cool research" that presents many similar problems.

The Problem with "Cool Research"

Breakthroughs are sought above all else within the academic publishing world. Therefore, there is a clear bias towards positive, exciting research which develops new treatments, and there is little appetite or money to independently rerun experiments to confirm or debunk initial results. It simply means that once a treatment is accepted, even if the scientific proof is iffy or nonexistent, it can be exceptionally difficult to stop its usage. Drug companies know this and are eager to get their drugs on the market as fast as possible (Remember: *Once the train has left the station…*). The FDA is complicit in this issue as well since money from the pharmaceutical industry is their major funding source.

Further, the drug industry has gone as far as to bury clinical trials when the results were negative. John Oliver, the host of the HBO series *Last Week Tonight with John Oliver*, did a brilliant, laugh-out-loud segment about this called "Scientific Studies."[11] After pointing out the frequent media misinterpretation of studies, he highlighted that the only way to verify that a study's results weren't a fluke was to redo the study, a replication study as they're called, which happens very infrequently. In the segment, Oliver shares the sentiments of scientist Dr. Elizabeth Iorns, who tells him, "[Replication studies] are rarely funded and so are underappreciated. There is no reward for doing them." Oliver sums it up after by saying "There is no Nobel Prize for fact checking."

Oncologist Vinay Prasad, author of more than 300 academic articles and the books *Ending Medical Reversal* and *Malignant*, concurs: "Medicine is quick to adopt practices based on shaky evidence but slow to drop them once they've been blown up by solid proof. We have a culture where we reward discovery; we don't reward replication."[12]

New positive research is more exciting; retesting initial scientific findings has low status. But considering the huge incentives for positive research, both at the university level and funded by Big Pharma, retesting is more crucial than ever.

The Problem with the "Smartest Doctors"

When I attended anesthesiology conferences, there were often panel discussions with experts in the field tackling thorny problems such as "Managing the Difficult Airway" or "Pediatric Pitfalls in Anesthesia." Anesthesiology is a field where practitioners can confront life-threatening clinical situations unexpectedly at any time during their shifts, so the more solutions and tools at their disposal, the better equipped they are at intervening effectively when a situation deteriorates. With this in mind, the expert panelists at these conferences often presented algorithms, decision trees and the latest science.

There would be a question-and-answer period following the panel discussion, and this was when I would pay the most attention. Often, doctors in the audience would stand up and offer how *they* had handled similar challenging situations. Some of these practitioners were in rural practices without access to help, let alone any cool toys; others were physicians in big county hospitals who were managing crisis after crisis and had to use what was on hand and fast. These doctors often had elegant, hard-won, practical solutions or "hacks" that I would tuck firmly into my memory.

There will always be a place of importance for the smartest people with the best training. And how could there not be? Smarter is better, right? But a bigger question is: What truly constitutes "smartness"? We usually think the doctor with the best degree is the "smartest," but there are limitations here. Does the doctor have repeated hands-on experience with a specific problem and a track record of positive results? Does the doctor carefully evaluate risk versus benefit?

This concept is age-old. While Aristotle believed in text-book learning, he emphasized *phronesis* or practical wisdom. This is the wisdom to clearly see what needs to be done and get it done, which can require years of experience to acquire. I often ended up deploying the strategies shared by the conference back-of-the-hall attendees when I needed fast, effective action. I also found that my colleague anesthesia nurse practitioners, who might not be considered the "smartest doctors" by stereotypical thinking, often had years of experience and were a rich source of practical solutions and sound judgement. They were ones with *phronesis*.

The Problem of Inadequate Mental Models: Man-as-Machine

Thinking of second and third-order consequences of your actions is difficult if your mental model is deficient or defective. While the body is a sophisticated system of multiple feedback systems that can lead to homeostasis, modern medicine often considers it a machine whose individual parts need fixing.

In this *man-as-machine* model, the thinking goes that *the machine needs something done to it;* otherwise, it will not get better. But this can lead to incorrect diagnosis and inaccurate treatment options. Remedies that seem logical according to this way of thinking do not necessarily work as intended, a pitfall *New York Times* bestselling author David Epstein dubbed *bio-plausibility*. In a nutshell, it refers to treatments that make logical sense to the physician but may not actually work.

Since the model of *man-as-machine* ignores the power of homeostatic feedback systems that can react to subtle inputs, it is difficult for many to believe that small changes or minor treatments can be enough. As such, the prevailing (and incorrect) attitude is that physical therapy, acupuncture, dietary changes and attention to sleeping habits hardly seem up to the challenge of serious problems.

The Problem of Perverse Incentives: How a Doctor's Thinking Gets Derailed

We've considered the pitfalls in relying on cool toys, cool research and smart doctors and how difficult it can be to do no harm. But there's something else we need to consider: the thought process of the physician. A doctor's thinking can become hopelessly derailed because of multiple perverse incentives as well as concerns over getting credit and blame—

and these derailments can be all-consuming. When doctors go astray, it usually happens in one of a few ways:

Conflicting Incentives

Conflicting incentives can lead to Dr. Twos becoming Dr. Threes. Just as we saw with drug companies wanting to get their undertested drugs onto the market or researchers rushing their half-baked findings to press, the incentives to treat and to be an *interventionista* are intense. Those pressures can come from wanting to please and retain patients to wanting a fat payday to wanting to avoid criticism from the medical community.

Pressure from Patients

On the other side, patients have a pronounced bias towards action and can apply subtle and not-so-subtle pressure to their doctors. They hear about a treatment or see a persuasive TV commercial and want it, even if it might not be appropriate for them. And if the patients push hard enough, doctors often give them what they want.

Follow the Money

The desire or need to make a profit exists at every level of our modern healthcare system. We've all heard stories about a single aspirin costing $30 in an emergency room. To treat is to make money. As Sinclair Lewis, the first American to win a Nobel Prize in Literature, eloquently said, "It is difficult to get a man to understand something when his salary depends upon his not understanding it." In this context, it is difficult to get a surgeon to stop doing a useless procedure when he makes his money doing it. A surgeon's first inclination is to do what he spent years learning to do: perform surgery. Consider this a version of the old adage, "To the hammer, everything looks like a nail." Similarly, expensive imaging machinery or medical devices (cool toys) need to be deployed to make the huge initial investment pay off.

Credit and Blame

Complicated medical conditions can involve complex treatment involving multiple specialists. In the end, no one may be really in charge, and so no one is accountable. The Bowie story is a classic example of this, as he had so many doctors. Once his stimulator was in and malfunctioning, no doctors were willing to take the chance at removal because no *one* doctor was in charge. Here, we see the opposite of the *interventionista* approach where not one of the physicians who participated in Bowie's tragic unraveling wanted to be blamed for causing a disastrous final result, of which there was a high likelihood. It took a doctor who had no expertise in stimulators at all (not *the smartest doctor*) to stand up. He took the risk to his reputation, possible recriminations from Bowie's family and the possibility of catastrophe to save Bowie's life.

When Evidence Says No, but Doctors Say Yes

Author David Epstein wrote a seminal article titled "When Evidence Says No, but Doctors Say Yes," a remarkable exposé of treatments that are broadly used but have little scientific substantiation. He wrote:

> *Years after research contradicts common practices, patients continue to demand them and doctors continue to deliver. The result is an epidemic of unnecessary and unhelpful treatment. When you visit a doctor, you probably assume the treatment you receive is backed by evidence from medical research. Surely, the drug you're prescribed or the surgery you'll undergo wouldn't be so common if it didn't work, right?* [13]

Well, we know this could very well not be right. Why? Because of the urgency of releasing medications without adequate vetting and procedures that have not been thoroughly evaluated for risks. Epstein goes on to state, "Some of the most widely prescribed medications do little of anything meaningful, good or bad, for most people who take them. So rather than waiting to prescribe or doing nothing, treatments are prescribed that do not confer huge improvements, rather they do nothing or worse."

Useless treatment is compounded by the fact that doctors will often not be faulted for taking this course of action (credit and blame). And if you add in the pursuit of profit (they will be leaving money on the table by not doing the procedure), it is a recipe for overtreatment and sometimes disaster. A Dr. One is committed to maintaining balance in his patients as the safest way to healing, and only when absolutely necessary does he resort to drastic intervention. As Gracián says, he acts as the wise physician who knows when not to prescribe. Unfortunately, our medical system is more likely to blame a doctor for *not* treating a patient than administering a treatment that ends up creating complications. As a result, it is often easier to be a Dr. Three than a Dr. One.

Epstein cites various examples of this situation. One is coronary artery stents, where a tube is inserted into a coronary artery to keep it open if it is clogged with plaque and causing disease:

Stenting is what scientists call "bio-plausible"—intuition suggests it should work. It's just that the human body is a little more Book of Job and a little less household plumbing: Humans didn't invent it, it's really complicated, and people often have remarkably little insight into cause and effect. Just as the cardiovascular system is not a kitchen sink [requiring roto rooter remedies], the musculoskeletal system is not an erector set. Cause and effect is frequently elusive.

Another example is arthroscopic partial meniscectomy (APM), which cleans out damaged tissue to alleviate knee pain and accounts for roughly a half-million yearly procedures. "This is not a fringe surgery," Epstein writes. "In recent years, it has been one of the most popular surgical procedures at a cost of around $4 billion."

But a burgeoning body of evidence says that APM *does not work* for the most common varieties of knee pain. Studies have shown that patients have the same relief whether they get surgery or not—as long as they get physical therapy. In an extremely rare "sham surgery" study from 2013, some patients got incisions but no surgery done on the meniscus as a control group while others had the real procedure. A year later, there was no difference in the results between the two groups—except that patients who had the real surgery were *more likely to develop osteoarthritis*.

How can a procedure so contraindicated by research be so common? Epstein got answers from surgeons. One told him, "Most of my colleagues will say: 'Look, save yourself the headache, just do the surgery. None of us are going to be upset with you for doing the surgery. Your bank account's not going to be upset with you for doing the surgery. Just do the surgery.'"

One would be hard-pressed to find a more revealing indictment of the perverse incentives laid bare in medical decision making, and yet the above is an account from an *actual surgeon.*

As shown by the above, there are many situations where Dr. Twos can morph into Dr. Threes who lead patients into unnecessary surgery and all its inherent risks. In the case of APM, the risk is an increased likelihood of osteoarthritis of the knee. In Micah Bowie's case, the risks were even more severe, which makes it all the more helpful to illustrate the challenges doctors can encounter that can lead to derailment.

Follow the Money

All of the options in front of Bowie came at a high cost. In the US, back surgery costs between $65,000 and $200,000, depending on the severity of the case and where you live. The quoted cost for spinal cord stimulators today is $57,896 with yearly maintenance somewhere between $5,000 and $21,000, depending on complications. Bowie spent more than $400,000 on his medical bills and care and was bankrupted by the treatment process.

Bio-Plausibility and Its Limitations

Bowie most likely had a definite problem that was visible on his X-rays—but once something is observed on an X-ray, both the patient and sadly the doctor tend to consider it to be beyond the body's ability to repair. For many ailments, the presence of a mass, tear or break on an X-ray means the diagnosis is more serious, though this is not necessarily the case with back pain.

Back pain of the nonspecific variety is common enough that we have decades of experience with treatment, imaging and diagnosis. One study examined the question, "In patients with nonspecific low back pain, do lumbar X-ray scans modify any patient outcome?" The researchers determined that X-ray scans did nothing to improve outcomes and might actually worsen some of them (such as pain), writing:

> *Because X-ray scans for nonspecific LBP increase physician workload, expose patients to very high doses of radiation, and might actually worsen short-term outcomes [at three months, patients with X-rays had significantly worse pain], many trials have been conducted to discourage this practice.*[14]

For these reasons, the UK's National Institute for Health

and Care Excellence (NICE) eliminated back X-rays for pain since they did not correlate with pain or disability.[15] This lack of correlation is tough to believe, because it just seems so *logical* and *plausible* that abnormalities on a patient's X-rays would mean their back pain was more serious and thus would require serious treatment.

Even though studies repeatedly show that factors that affect back pain include mental state, depression and stress, problematic X-rays can still tilt patients into Dr. Three's office. Remember that Bowie showed tears associated with his fourth and fifth lumbar vertebrae and was having no luck controlling the pain, with the only solution on the horizon being repeated back surgeries. With this distressing prospect in mind, he opted for the "cool toy" of spinal cord stimulation and deteriorated from there.

Incentives, Credit and Blame

Because of the many layers of treatment Bowie received, there appeared to be no single decision-maker. This lack of accountability became challenging as the case continued and became disastrous, and no one wanted to take responsibility. As the saying goes, "Success has many fathers; failure is an orphan."

Smartest Doctors

In a last-ditch effort to get relief from the malfunctioning new device, Bowie went to a famous clinic with the "smartest doctors", but even there, the doctors were out of their depth faced with a novel type of injury. Bowie was spiraling out of control and none of the doctors wanted to be responsible for his downfall (*credit and blame*), so they advised him to "get his affairs in order." Out of desperation, Bowie turned to his previous groin surgeon and found in him someone willing to be accountable and face criticism, which saved Bowie's life. As Bowie's story shows, to be a Dr. One is not all that easy, and sometimes being a Dr. Two isn't either. It requires wisdom and resistance to pressure.

Avoidance Tactics Can Lead to Better Outcomes

Avoidance is clearly one of the pillars of staying healthy to escape needless harm, and it might have been easier for a Dr. One to achieve in ancient times—partly because there were fewer remedies, but also because of a better alignment of incentives around accountability, credit and blame. Dr. One held himself accountable for keeping his patients well. His way to do this was not in seeking dramatic treatment as his most powerful tool, let alone a way to make money. His model was not "fee for service" but rather "fee for health." Also, presumably, no established industries were putting pressure on physicians to treat as Big Pharma does today.

We cannot know for sure, but because this teaching still exists, we can surmise that ancient doctors garnered recognition if their patients remained well and were able to withstand illness and injury. This is near impossible in today's world where few accountable doctors or entities exist. Accountability is dispersed through different specialists and therapists. Consider a patient taking 10 or more medications prescribed by various specialists. Sometimes those medications can interact with each other, causing symptoms that require *more* prescriptions, and those negative interactions can be overlooked or missed when so many separate practitioners are involved in a treatment plan. The result can be a vicious downward spiral that leads to serious health problems.

More Is Not Always More

One of the frustrating things about public health measures like sanitation or personal health measures like diet and exercise is that they are so uncool and undramatic that there is no glory in them. But these are the very methods that *should* receive more funding. These measures are the essence of avoiding harm! Providing healthy food in poverty-stricken neighborhoods and facilities and green spaces at low cost for exercising could be beneficial and life-saving! But when we do them, no one gets to ride in on a white (and preferably robotic) horse to save the day.

In Bowie's case, doing "more" did *not* include the most invasive intervention, which would have been spinal surgery. But it did include the most recent, specialized and "coolest" intervention. It is highly likely that Bowie would have felt that he was not being listened to if the doctors had recommended a treatment pause, or acupuncture, physical therapy or vacation. He needed *big help*, so there was no time to allow for small measures or for homeostasis to play a role. In a sense, trying to be a Dr. One in Bowie's case would have been ineffectual, as he might've simply sought help elsewhere.

The truth is it is difficult for us to believe that small changes or minor treatments can be "enough," especially when it comes to pain. All-too-natural reactions from 21st century patients are along the lines of: "No! This pain is really, really bad! I need to get rid of it! I need strong medication! I need the latest and the greatest!"

Pain is not only debilitating but also depressing and terrifying (which we will discuss at length in Chapter Seven), but we must keep in mind that we need balance and small stressors for everything to "spin together," especially with an issue like Bowie's back pain. As human beings, this approach does not seem rational or proportional to us. But we must abandon the expectation that proportionality is always warranted.

Sometimes, small actions are required and sometimes nothing is required. This is probably one of the hardest mental models to embrace, though it is also one of the most important.

But What If...?

Hindsight is 20/20, of course, but what if Bowie's doctors had considered more options? *What if* he was given options for acupuncture, massage, gradual physical therapy, stress reduction or a spa vacation? Clearly, he had a serious problem, *but what if* the thinking and mental models allowed another strategy to be a valid choice? Could he have had a different outcome?

Alternative measures may not have been enough, but there would have been minimal harm in trying them. We will never know with Bowie, but stories like his should open our thinking to consider, if not embrace, other mental models. The *what if* discussions can make us uncomfortable and even cringe, as we know and appreciate that doctors work their hearts out and do not want to blame them. They confront profound challenges and do heroic work. As a medical doctor —both a board-certified pediatrician and anesthesiologist—I take the real problems of decision-making seriously. It is hard enough in the best of times, and when faced with so many pitfalls, it can be nearly impossible to do well. But we must keep the real goal in mind: to stay healthy and reduce harm in the face of the powerful forces that work against that principle. This is the promise and challenge of Dr. One's philosophy.

Chapter 3
Your Stress Response: The Deep Power of Balance

"Stress is not a state of mind...it's measurable and dangerous and humans can't seem to find their off switch."
–Robert Sapolsky, PhD, *Why Zebras Don't Get Ulcers*[1]

A Stranger in a Strange Land: A Student Abroad

For a year, at age 17, I was an exchange student living in Zurich, Switzerland. Within a short time of settling in with my host family, I was suddenly ravenous, constantly craving food. I developed an ugly case of acne, which was the last thing I needed when trying to meet new people in a foreign country. I either could not sleep or slept too much. Looking at photos of myself during that year, I am unrecognizable. My skinny ballerina frame had thickened. My face looked like I was storing nuts in my cheeks. What happened to me? Logic might tell you that the delicious Swiss chocolate and tempting ever-present sausages were to blame, but that would be wrong. There was much more to it than that.

From the outside, my student exchange year in Switzerland might sound idyllic: a kid is transplanted to a beautiful, prosperous European city courtesy of an American Field

Service (AFS) scholarship. What an opportunity and what an experience! But consider this: I was a teenager, still a child in many respects, who only knew my family, home and friends in Northern California (radical Berkeley, no less), which was a far cry from the reserved, conservative world of 1970s Switzerland.

Whatever its undoubted positive attributes, Zurich was still a foreign environment, and this was decades before cell phones or the internet. At the time, there was no meaningful way to communicate with family and friends back home. Instead of a large, integrated, raucous, co-ed public high school, I was at a buttoned-up, all-girls school. I looked dramatically different from my classmates and was a stranger in a strange land.

The goal of the AFS exchange was total immersion in a new family to ensure that students got the most out of the experience. That meant no phone calls, packages or funds from home were allowed, only letters. Furthermore, AFS instructed host families to only speak in the host country's language. Though I was a teenager who desperately wanted friends, music and fun, I couldn't communicate. Not only did I not know German (five years of High School French, thank you very much), but when not in class, my peers spoke Swiss German, which was yet another language. To my classmates, I seemed like a backward child who could not understand their jokes, and it was impossible to convince them how cool I was. I was alone, homesick, and desperate to learn German. Though I was a teenager in a civilized city who should've had no cares in the world, my entire body spiraled out of control because of the *interpretation* of my experience. It was all because of stress.

When Mind Affects Body

Before I continue, let me say that this story is not in any way comparable to the most horrendous and extreme stress experienced by much of humanity, but I only use it to illustrate how damaging and extreme stress can become even in relatively "mild" situations. Similarly, not everyone reading this may be in actual life-or-death situations every day, but their bodies and health may still be out of balance as a result of chronic stress for all kinds of reasons.

In Switzerland, I was a fish out of water. My new life required constant studying, learning German and trying to show my peers that I was not foreign, not other. As humans, we are tribal. For our primitive selves, an expulsion from the tribe meant death, so it is not surprising that fear of ridicule or ostracism is deeply ingrained in our nervous systems. When I experienced it as a teen, my body reacted to that unrelenting stress and became chronically unbalanced.

To be fair to my younger self, teenagers suffer terribly from this phantom stress of being uncool, shunned or not belonging. It can lead to the ultimate spiraling out of control—suicide, a leading killer of teens. Horrifically, 24-hour-a-day internet and social media have added to our stress, especially for young people. Just when you need to have high-quality sleep to perform in school and face everyday challenges, the overabundance of stress-induced cortisol and adrenaline coursing through your body can wreck it and degrade your mood even more. In the modern "first world," many of our threats are virtual. The point of my Switzerland story, then, is that threats—even phantom ones—can still wreak havoc on our systems. It's a unique human condition.

In retrospect, I have no doubt that I had elevated cortisol in Switzerland, which was a safe situation. With that in mind, we can extrapolate the effects of stress to people like refugees, teenage army recruits or young people living in precarious neighborhoods in the US. You can see how stress can affect everything and cause all sorts of damage.

In my case, I was lucky. I started to feel better in the last month of my stay. Knowing I would soon be home, my skin cleared. The physical changes were transitory and the overall experience perhaps made me stronger or at least better at studying. But others aren't so lucky; it all depends on how capable our bodies are at managing stress.

What Doesn't Kill You Does Not Always Make You Stronger

How our body responds to stress affects so many aspects of our health. Elevated stress can adversely affect our health, compounding every condition covered in this book. Stress is a multi-faceted threat that illustrates the importance of Dr. One's strategies of maintaining balance by avoiding harm and introducing hormetic challenges.

The stress response constantly maintains balance and homeostasis to keep everything running smoothly. However, as with many feedback systems, the stress response can also go haywire and hurt us even though it aims to help us. In the struggle against adversity, the trope that "what doesn't kill you makes you stronger" is *not* correct when stress is relentless. Unfortunately, for people who live in poverty, war-torn countries or any situation where stress is constant, their bodies can sustain lasting damage.

Chronic stress can affect the brain, putting the parts that deal with danger in overdrive. Meanwhile, the other parts of the brain that deal with memory, planning and other higher functions become starved of resources. In turn, this can lead to more acute *and* long-term stress, potentially creating "faulty wiring" in the brain and creating a downward spiral. So, managing this important system is a potent tool for measuring and maintaining balance in a modern-day Dr. One's medicine bag.

How the Stress Response Works to Save You: Fast and Slow

The two key aspects of the stress response, our body's reaction to attack, are the autonomic nervous system and the hypothalamic-pituitary-adrenal axis. Stanford University professor, primatologist and author Robert Sapolsky likens the instantaneous response of the autonomic nervous system to handing out machine guns in the face of an attack. Meanwhile, the hypothalamic–pituitary–adrenal axis is more like building aircraft carriers for long-haul effort. Let's look at each one separately.

The Autonomic Nervous System: Fast Stress Responses

The autonomic nervous system is *automatic.* It functions without our mind's input, as an involuntary reflex process. Part of the autonomic nervous system is **the sympathetic nervous system**, the primitive fight-or-flight reflex, which is our savior when we are under acute attack. In these situations, the restorative, longer-term concerns of the **parasympathetic nervous system** are put on hold, enabling us to live another day.

The Sympathetic Branch of the Autonomic Nervous System: Fight, Flee, Freeze

The fight-or-flight reflex leads to adrenaline surges. In defiance of its name, is not prone to taking the time for sympathy. It is fight or run for your life, a hardwired evolutionary response that gives you that racing heart at the unexpected bark of a nearby dog, the threat of a fall or during a testy conversation with your boss. It gives you butterflies in your stomach and cold hands when speaking in public.

By stimulating rapid heartbeat, dilated pupils and higher blood pressure, we are better able to either flee or stay and fight. Energy resources pour into our muscles and away from other essential activities such as digestion or immune function. After all, fighting off a cold or digesting lunch can wait until you are safely up that tree.

The Parasympathetic Branch of the Autonomic Nervous System: Rest, Digest, Regroup

Parasympathetic activity is essential for building, restoring, healing and sleeping. It relies on the lengthy vagus nerve that extends from the brain's medulla to the intestines. It is involved in heart, gastrointestinal, immune and endocrine functions. The Latin word *vagus* means "wandering," and the words "vagrant" and "vagabond" come from the same root.

As the vagus nerve has tentacles everywhere, its sensing fibers can detect a wide array of inputs—pressure, pain, stretch, temperature, chemicals and inflammation. The "gut feelings" that we experience may well rely on these primitive inputs that bypass the brain. In fact, the gut is called "the second brain" because of the tight association between vagal activity and these vast unconscious inputs. The vagus is also involved in the homeostasis of the digestive tract and the generation of heart and respiratory rhythms.

The Hypothalamic-Pituitary-Adrenal Axis: Slow Stress Response Where Cortisol Reigns

The main agent of hypothalamic–pituitary–adrenal axis (a long, complicated name for the slower aspect of the stress response) is the steroid hormone cortisol. Three intercommunicating regions of the body mainly control the secretion of cortisol: the hypothalamus in the brain, the pituitary gland and the adrenal gland—hence the hypothalamic–pituitary–adrenal axis.

Because this system is a hormone-driven response, it is slower to act. Cortisol is released from the adrenal gland after the release of adrenaline and stays around longer. It binds to almost all body cells and leads to a decrease in immune response, alterations in glucose metabolism and other effects that aim to increase energy resources to fend off an attack. The effect of cortisol is to stimulate fat and carbohydrate metabolism for fast energy sources.

When prolonged, the result of these actions can be an increase in appetite and cravings for sweet, high-fat and salty foods. The result? Weight gain as a means of survival. Cortisol can also result in insomnia, because it is a main driver of daily rhythms and can spike at night. On top of that, it can exacerbate many skin conditions, especially acne.

Measuring cortisol would be one way to monitor the stress response. Indeed, many studies on stress include cortisol as a biomarker. But it is part of the slow response. A more immediate means to measure stress is through the fast-responding autonomic nervous system. One way to measure autonomic balance on a second-by-second basis is through monitoring what could be called the flexibility of the heart, or how well the heart reacts to challenges. The heart is influenced by both arms of the autonomic nervous system, the parasympathetic and sympathetic. We can measure relative inputs from both by looking at the variability in heart rhythm.

Heart Rate Variability Measures Autonomic Balance: Seeing the Unseen

When I started my acupuncture practice, the nagging question in the back of my mind was exactly how acupuncture cured my allergies. The scientific hypothesis for how acupuncture worked at the time was through "gating," a process whereby needles occupied nerve endings. As a result, pain impulses could not reach the brain. But gating could not explain the disappearance of my allergies.

By chance, I heard a talk by Robert Sapolsky, who focused on the adverse effects of stress on many of the body's functions, including the immune system. This talk got me thinking about my allergies. Dr. Sapolsky explained that our systems did not evolve for repeated or prolonged stress; they could tip into *too much* immunity, with our bodies attacking our own tissues as a result. This is the phenomenon of autoimmunity. Because allergies are one type of autoimmunity, perhaps somehow acupuncture altered my stress levels and helped my system stop attacking itself, causing my allergies to diminish.

As an anesthesiologist, I embraced the idea of monitoring patients during their acupuncture treatments. After some searching, I found a monitoring method called heart rate variability (HRV), which uses complex computer analysis of heart rate variation with breathing to measure the balance between the sympathetic and parasympathetic nervous systems.

Why Variability Means Stability—and Uniformity Means Death

The ancients knew the significance of heart rate variability. In the third century, Wang-Shu Ho, wrote, "If the pattern of the heartbeat becomes as regular as the tapping of a woodpecker or the dripping of rain from the roof, the patient will be dead in four days." The internal physics of the lungs expanding against the heart within its pericardium, the innervation of the heart via the vagus and the rush of adrenaline all contribute to making heart rate variability a complex measurement. Through measuring these subtle forces on the heart, we can infer the overall balance in the autonomic nervous system, which, in turn, exerts its effects on the body's many feedback systems.

Variability of heart rate within certain bounds is a sign of health. We see this variability not only in heart rate but in other physical measurements, such as a person's gait. Variability is a healthy feature because it means the stresses on the heart are more evenly spread and not repeatedly inflicted on one particular part. This shows nature's wisdom in designing the heart.

Jay Harmon, the biomimicry scientist and engineer, says, "No man-made pump and piping can match the efficiency of the human heart and vascular system." But this natural variability decreases with age, injury or depression. Stress also reduces heart rate variability because of the increase in fight-or-flight autonomic activity and a decrease in rest-and-digest. What makes the heart more human, the lovely variability, becomes more machinelike with challenges to the body.

The real advantage of monitoring heart rate variability (HRV) for the clinician or researcher is that it can be used at the bedside. Better yet, it is noninvasive and doesn't interfere with treatment. We can get a snapshot of autonomic balance or stress levels at a specific moment in time, or we can also monitor HRV over a longer period as well. We can use HRV to assess the effect of treatment, thereby *making the invisible visible*. HRV monitoring is something I regularly use in my practice, and it was particularly helpful during acupuncture treatments with a patient I'll call Teresa.

Teresa's Story

I used my new heart rate variability (HRV) monitoring system when I treated Teresa, a young mother with three children under the age of four. She was an athlete and a writer and was hale and hearty, educated, energetic and fun. But she had panic attacks when driving on freeways that got even worse when she had to cross a bridge. She'd tried cognitive behavioral therapy (CBT) to no avail. She did not want to take tranquilizers because she needed to be able to drive and work. She knew her fear was nonsense, but it was taking over her life.

Teresa exhibited typical panic attack symptoms: queasiness and pain in her stomach followed by a rapid heart rate, discomfort, and a sense her throat was closing. This can be terrifying for patients, as they truly feel like they might be dying. I recognized that this constellation of symptoms was similar to a syndrome in Chinese medicine called "running piglet." The "piglet" is running the wrong way in one of the special meridians of the body, wreaking havoc. The condition has a specific needling protocol which I used on Teresa, and after only three acupuncture treatments, there was rapid and remarkable improvement and fewer panic attacks. It was a dramatic and decisive success. Teresa continued regular treatment and tapered off after the attacks stopped.

The HRV monitoring system data provided one of the keys to the puzzle of stress, acupuncture and perhaps how it had helped Teresa. I measured her HRV during needling and then while she was resting with needles in place. I began looking for patterns, not knowing what I would find. My "aha" moment came when I noticed that Teresa's heart rate variability tracings spiked in her sympathetic fight-or-flight output during needling, followed by a decline below baseline. In other words, her result showed a decrease in autonomic nervous system stress response (a "relaxation response") on the table after needling. When I compared Teresa to other patients, this pronounced decrease in autonomic nervous system stress response was characteristic of patients who responded well and promptly to acupuncture treatment. This decrease did not occur in those who did not respond.

I wrote up this observation and had it published in the *Journal of Medical Acupuncture*, but I knew my observational findings needed further validation.[2] Within months of publication, a German acupuncture study described similar results in a group of migraine patients.[3] Those who showed decreased fight-or-flight during acupuncture also had a reduction in their migraines. I had so many questions about what exactly that correlation meant. Was it making patients more resilient? Was it a sign that certain patients are more "flexible" and more susceptible to treatment? Could the results depend on the exact needling protocol that was used? If that were the case, could changing the needling protocol lead to a better reduction in their stress response?

With so many unanswered questions, I knew that HRV monitoring would be something I would keep using as an adjunct to acupuncture treatment.

Acupuncture Treatment and the Stress Response: Stoking the Flywheel

The temporary increase in stress levels immediately upon needling shows the body's reaction to the procedure. We now know it sets off cascades of responses not only in the autonomic nervous system but also in pain circuits, immune responses and other homeostatic systems. It sets the system spinning like a flywheel of positive responses.

Research shows that the minor challenge of acupuncture needles decreases stress, which correlates with an increase in resilience. This translates into toughness in the face of physiologic or emotional challenges. It's difficult to know how long this resilience might last after treatment, but animal studies provide clues.

Two recent studies looked at the effect of acupuncture on the stress response reactions of beagles and horses. In the dog study, after receiving acupuncture, a group of beagles were challenged with a recording of thunder, a clever intervention which was harmless to the dogs but put them in a state of high alert and sympathetic overdrive.[4] The acupuncture session reduced the spike in sympathetic fight-or-flight activity compared with a control group of beagles who did not get acupuncture. But the acupuncture also decreased their physical reactions—hiding, restlessness, bolting and running around.

Similarly, the horse study found that acupuncture reduced the spike in sympathetic fight-or-flight activity when they were startled by the opening of an umbrella near their heads (another safe and cunning way to "stress" the horses without harming them).[5]

These findings are quite remarkable and give us a key to Dr. One's strategy for maintaining balance in his patients. We learn that treatment with acupuncture can stabilize this autonomic response and limit spiraling out of control.

These fight-or-flight reactions to challenges occur in humans too. Even a temporary spike in sympathetic activity sometimes leads to impaired performance, poor judgment or a hypervigilant, fragile state. Used proactively, acupuncture can be beneficial. A study with athletes, for instance, found that acupuncture before a competitive event led to less anxiety and improved confidence and performance.[6]

Again, how is this possible? How can this minor intervention of needling stimulate such a profound bodily change? I credit the leverage of the many feedback systems of radical prevention that the good Dr. One knows. More is not always more, and small changes can produce outsized results as good systems biologists are well aware.

Systems Biology Meets Complexity Science: Measuring Resilience

Acupuncture and other complementary medical interventions can be better understood through the recent field of systems biology. In systems biology, scientists study the patterns that arise from *the interaction of multiple individual parts*. A single impetus can set off a web or cascade of reactions, not just a linear chain of events. Think of it like a mobile, and how a slight touch can cause the entire mobile to move before finding equilibrium again. Or consider Jay Harman's tiny turbine from Chapter 1 that spins and circulates a huge reservoir of liquid.

These interactions require a complex style of measurement that borrows from a range of disciplines including physics and engineering and others. These networks of multiple simple parts allow feed-forward loops and feedback loops. What is important to understand here is that output is not proportional to the input; a small perturbation can have large and sometimes unpredictable effects.

Systems biology can help us better understand this as we start to look at global behavior rather than one particular variable. It becomes possible to imagine measuring Dr. One's goal of "balance" as a global state. In complexity science, this state of balance can be measured as "adaptability" or "robustness." Through these feed-forward loops, we might see a gradual improvement in, say, allergic response. But this framework can allow for a sudden outsized change in allergic response too. To do this quantitatively requires complex computational tools borrowed from linear algebra, differential calculus, statistics, information theory or computational science. The measurement of heart rate variability (HRV) borrows from all these disciplines.

Through research, we've seen that improved HRV may indicate a patient is responding favorably to acupuncture. The question then becomes, "Could we use HRV to measure balance or 'robustness' in conjunction with acupuncture?" By doing so, we could make Dr. One's goal of "balance" as prevention measurable.

Can Acupuncture Improve HRV over Time?

We saw that acupuncture in beagles, horses and human athletes can stabilize the body for as long as minutes to hours after treatment. But what about a longer period of weeks to months? Because blood pressure is measurable by conventional means, Stanford anesthesiologist Dr. Brenda Golianu and I studied HRV in hypertensive patients over weeks to months. We found that blood pressure and sympathetic flight-or-fight activity decreased over the study period in patients who responded to acupuncture.[7] Researchers led by Puja K. Mehta confirmed these findings in patients with coronary artery disease, who with consistent acupuncture had a decrease in fight-or-flight over months, along with a parallel reduction in biomarkers for coronary artery disease.[8]

A decrease in stress levels is more significant than you might think because of the way our feedback systems work. Enabling patients with hypertension to jettison just one medication can improve their lives because they are likely to have fewer side effects. In addition, lowering stress levels has positive effects on virtually every system in the body (as we will see in Chapter 5, increasing rest-and-digest or vagal activity in lab animals after acupuncture treatment led to increased survival of the severe infection phenomenon of sepsis[9]). Using the tools of complexity science to measure biomarker outcomes such as HRV, we may be able to quantify the balance that Dr. One seeks.

How the Body Affects the Mind

But what about the third pillar of Dr. One? How does this all spin together? How can this balance work for prevention? We've seen some clues, but let's reflect on my patient Teresa. How do we explain Teresa's prompt response to treatment? As with many patients battling panic attacks, it is often *unconscious body reactions* that generate an exaggerated fight-or-flight response. It may be the downside of our second brain, the gut, that senses something without our awareness.

Once the attack starts, however, the mind leaps into action, trying to find an explanation. The experience— thoughts of *I'm dying, I'm dying*—is so vivid and intense for the person that it can be impossible to talk themselves down. Thoughts racing out of control can perpetuate their distress and land them in the emergency room. Even *worrying about* a triggering event can cause a full-blown panic attack for these patients.

In Teresa's situation, the acupuncture might simply have calmed her body, just as it worked for the beagles, horses and athletes. The body becomes sturdier and more resilient by treatment with acupuncture, so it has fewer unconscious fight-or-flight reactions. This stability and balance is the dominion of Dr. One, and leads to prevention and radical resilience.

It would be helpful to have a way to show this type of resilience so that even in the absence of symptoms to track, you could measure progress or deterioration. This is yet another potential way to use HRV to measure the intangible, and one that follows the philosophy of Dr. One.

Measuring "Well-Being"

How do we measure a person's overall state, such as "well-being" or "health"? If we think about it, that really is what we're looking for when we seek out medical help. Studies comparing HRV with overall health, well-being and even the likelihood of contracting non-contagious disease suggest that HRV may correlate with resilience, as researchers in systems biology and complexity science hypothesized.[10] As such, researchers have noted that HRV may be a good way to measure many different difficult-to-measure things like health, well-being, adaptability and resilience.

Radical Resilience

According to the authors of an article in Complementary and Alternative Medicine (CAM), "The capacity to capture the global state of a system or an individual suggests these complexity-based measures (such as heart rate variability) may act as surrogates for concepts that were traditionally difficult to measure but considered important for Complementary and Alternative Medicine (CAM) research (e.g., "health" and "adaptability")."[11] Thus, a complex measurement like HRV can give an overview of these complex systems that are interacting to produce an overall state like "well-being," "adaptability" or "resilience" as an actual measurement.

One research group interested in what would most closely correlate with "self-rated health," or *how healthy* patients themselves felt they were, looked at HRV and other measures of health, such as inflammatory markers.[12] They found that HRV correlated the closest, and that all measures of autonomic nervous system function were significantly more strongly associated with self-rated health than any other measure. The rather "fuzzy" concept of health has become quantifiable, and the invisible is now visible. This is important because HRV may be a way to evaluate the body's resilience and improve it *even when healthy*, improving sturdiness and providing radical prevention.

The authors of another recent HRV study say it "has emerged as a physiological indicator for emotional regulation and psychological well-being."[13] In clinical populations of either depression or anxiety, HRV was *lower,* indicating *more* fight-or-flight stress levels compared to controls.

An article in the *Journal of Clinical Medicine* points to HRV as a public health predictor of noncommunicable (non-infectious) disease, highlighting the tight association of parasympathetic rest-and-digest activity with the ability to lessen the behavioral factors that contribute to diseases which are the big killers: cardiovascular disease, cancer and lung disease.[14] The group seeks to introduce "a new paradigm to predict, understand, prevent and possibly treat such diseases based on the science of neuro-immunology and specifically by focusing on vagal neuro-modulation." This group advocates monitoring HRV and implementing vagal nerve stimulation as a therapy, though it is worth noting that *acupuncture can achieve similar ends.*

Vagal nerve activity is related to frontal brain activity, which regulates unhealthy lifestyle behaviors. If you have higher parasympathetic activity, you are more likely to be able to control unhealthy behaviors and institute healthy ones. The vagus nerve acts as a sort of go-between linking the portion of the brain which helps control behavior with physiological states.

The authors explain that epidemiologically, high vagal activity, shown by greater heart rate variability, independently predicts better prognosis and reduced risk of diseases.

The Prevention of the Future: How HRV Can Measure the Balance Sought by Dr. One

Heart rate variability (HRV) is a modern tool to monitor an ancient concept of balance which can foster deep resilience. As the studies show, if you improve parasympathetic activity, it not only enhances health from a physical standpoint but also encourages healthy habits. Because of the tight mind-body connection, this leads to an overall health condition we call well-being.

There will always be a role for medications, joint replacements and trauma surgery, but the "moonshot" is to be able to trigger and harness our feedback systems and avoid harm— thus becoming more resilient to disease, achieving a healthy lifestyle and living longer. By learning smarter ways to do this, we stay tougher and more resistant to spiraling out of control.

We need more research into how we can make acupuncture more effective and more reliable (like gravity). We are making progress, and the potential could be substantial. It may be that more is more, namely that more frequent acupuncture would help stabilize the system more. But other qualities may also be more critical. Keep in mind that medicine, in general, is not like gravity. It doesn't follow the hard and fast rules of physics. As one of the fathers of modern medicine, William Osler, once said, "Medicine is a science of uncertainty and the art of probability." The body is a system of feedbacks, not a machine. Ideally, our methods of treatment and measurement of outcomes should reflect this system approach.

Bio monitors like HRV may be well suited to develop and measure a new kind of balance and toughness and to develop better treatment strategies. Since there are many challenges in modern life—pollutants, upheaval, food contamination and epidemics, for instance—rather than finding specific means to counter every challenge, we start to create the prevention of the future by fostering overall resilience in the individual.

Systems Synergy and How "It All Spins Together"

In this chapter, we have looked at how the stress response can affect the mind-body interaction. By decreasing fight-or-flight responses and increasing rest-and-digest responses, we can affect multiple systems in the body ranging from immunity and inflammation to mood and pain. While these conditions may not sound life-threatening to you, they are involved in cancer and heart disease that are killers. We will revisit this most crucial feedback system, the autonomic nervous system, throughout the book seeing how it wields its deep power.

Chapter 4
Longevity: Unlocking Our Cells' Secrets to Defy Aging

"Ad me'ah ve'esrim shanah (May you live until 120)."
—Hebrew blessing

Sandra's Story

Sandra was an attractive, petite woman in her late 30s who came to see me for anxiety and fertility issues after breaking up a vicious fight between two large dogs at the doggy daycare she ran. The danger, noise and chaos had riled up the other dogs and terrified Sandra and her staff, but Sandra was the most affected as she had fearlessly jumped in to separate the dogs.

Within two days of this dramatic dog fight, her hormonal profile showed that she was precipitously veering towards menopause. Modern medical doctors would probably write this off to chance, thinking that the sudden decline in her hormones would have happened anyway—but I knew Chinese medical practitioners might well explain this sudden onset of menopause as the logical result of a deep fright having affected Sandra's kidneys. As a construct in Chinese medicine, the kidneys do more than filter and remove waste. They are critical to the overall constitution and other functions, closely linked to the *jing* or "essence."

My task was to calm Sandra's nervous system and nourish her kidneys as best as possible, since her deepest desire was to have children. I used acupuncture point prescriptions to nourish her kidneys, especially her kidney *jing*. I also added in herbal treatments especially formulated for older mothers and saw her twice weekly. Notably, after two months of treatment Sandra became pregnant.

So, in a chapter about longevity, why am I bringing up this case? What do fertility and fear have to do with our desire to live longer? We will see how they connect when we tackle the concept of *jing* in more detail, but first, let us set our sights on our real end goal: not just to live long but to live with as much *life* as possible until the end. Longevity scientists emphasize that we seek a long "health span" rather than lifespan alone, as no one is inspired by the thought of living a long time but with an awful quality of life. The goal of medicine and prevention should be to allow for this possibility, and in this chapter, we'll explore how.

We will see how acupuncture leverages cellular responses that are key to longevity. We know that stress can lead to a deterioration in health and shorten telomeres, a measure of longevity. But the mechanisms triggered by acupuncture go beyond that system to include some of the recently discovered cellular mechanisms involved in aging, mimicking "health hacks" known to be good for longevity and metabolic health. These include practices such as calorie restriction, saunas, cold exposure, and more. We will see how one particular herb, renowned in Chinese medicine for longevity effects, also triggers these crucial cellular responses.

The Eternal Quest for the Fountain of Youth

The human interest in how long we can live has been with us for millennia. Consider this passage from *The Yellow Emperor's Classic of Medicine* published in the third millennium BCE:

> *I've heard that in the days of old, everyone lived one hundred years without showing the usual signs of aging. In our time, however, people age prematurely, living only fifty years. Is this due to a change in environment, or is it because people have lost the correct way of life?*

> *Qi Bo replied, "In the past, people practiced the Tao, the Way of Life. They understood the principle of balance, of yin and yang, as represented by the transformation of the energies of the universe. Thus, they formulated practices such as Dao-in, an exercise combining stretching, massaging, and breathing to promote energy flow, and meditation to help maintain and harmonize themselves with the universe. They ate a balanced diet at regular times, arose and retired at regular hours, avoided overstressing their bodies and minds, and refrained from overindulgence of all kinds. They maintained well-being of body and mind: thus it is not surprising that they lived over one hundred years.*[1]

In Ancient Chinese medicine, living 120 years was not regarded as unusual. Furthermore, 120 years seems to resonate across cultures and ages, as in the Hebrew blessing that serves as this chapter's epigraph. Science now shows that the neurons in our brains, unlike other cells in our bodies, can live up to 120 years—another instance of *modern eyes, ancient teachings.* Keeping that in mind, let's look at how the ancients understood aging and longevity before taking a tour of the modern science of aging that supports it.

The Ancient Concept of *Jing:* The Key to Longevity

In Chinese medicine, longevity is linked to a concept called *jing*, or essence, our primal life force. People lucky enough to be born with an abundance of *jing* will most likely be healthy, strong, resilient and achieve great longevity. When *jing* is abundant, as in a healthy newborn, it is like having a fully charged battery.

We all have our own allotment of *jing*. Though we can limit the leakage and recharge it with healthy, balanced living, nature dictates life and will eventually run it down, as with any battery. All minor or major disease diminishes *jing*, making us more susceptible to disease, degeneration and aging—all part of a vicious cycle and a classic example of spiraling out of control.

All death is ultimately associated with the loss of *jing*. As you read on, we will look at strategies to harness the body's longevity genes or nourish *jing* safely. But first, let us consider what the ancients called "anterior heaven" and "posterior heaven"—two concepts we know in modern medicine as genetics and epigenetics.

The Ancient Concepts of Anterior and Posterior Heaven: Genetics and Epigenetics

According to the ancient teachings, what you are born with—your potential—is your anterior heaven. You cannot control your anterior heaven; it is just the luck of the draw, your genetic inheritance. Conversely, posterior heaven represents your life circumstances and habits, and it can be affected by your health practices and how you live. But even with excellent anterior heaven and *jing*, if you are born into a situation of severe stress or malnutrition (a poor posterior heaven), you will eventually suffer health challenges and have a shortened life span.

Alternatively, even if you were born into royalty, for instance, and had hemophilia (like the last Russian Tsarevich, Alexei Nikolaevich), there would be limited options for this unlucky anterior heaven. No amount of right living would change it. But those who are born healthy, live wisely and guard their *jing* can theoretically live a very long time—even to 120 years. Of course, to fully take advantage of this potential requires some radical resilience. So, how do we get it?

The Modern Science of Aging

In recent years, with advances in microbiology and our ability to measure the body's most subtle inner workings, we have a clearer picture of why we age. By measuring some of these processes, we can devise strategies to prolong our health into old age.

Some ancient wisdom is now measurable, thanks to the modern eyes of science making the invisible visible. Modern advancements now provide us with tools and insights to objectively measure the effectiveness and relevance of ancient knowledge. Let's start with telomeres, a measure of potential longevity.

Telomeres: A Measure of Your Battery's Charge or *Jing*

A famous foray into the science of aging comes from the Nobel Prize-winning work of biological researcher Dr. Elizabeth Blackburn. She explored the science of telomeres, the segments of repeating DNA sequences at the end of our chromosomes, part of our genetic material. Telomeres protect the ends of chromosomes from deterioration or fusion with neighboring chromosomes. They are like the stiff endings that keep shoelaces from fraying. Telomere length measures potential longevity, and they get shorter as we age. In a groundbreaking study, Dr. Blackburn and her team found that telomeres also shorten under prolonged stress. [2]

Dr. Blackburn's researchers discovered that mothers of chronically ill children had shorter telomeres than mothers of healthy children. Though this had always been intuitively believed ("stress kills," after all), there had never been a measure of aging on the cellular level before to substantiate this belief. As her team showed, the imbalance of the autonomic nervous system caused by too much fight-or-flight and not enough rest-and-digest and its subsequent increases in cortisol can shorten your life. Put another way, stress can damage your posterior heaven.

In Sandra's case, we can see the dramatic consequences of experiencing a one-time, profound fright—but for the mothers in the study, it was an ongoing challenge and stress that led to shorter telomeres. [3] We know that a preponderance of fight-or-flight activity can lead to increased inflammation and poor immunity, provoking serious illnesses such as cardiovascular disease, cancer and potentially death. As such, the Yellow Emperor's admonition to live in moderation and to avoid "overstressing the body" is reinforced by the science of cell biology and telomeres. But there are also other players in the quest for longevity at a cellular level, as we'll soon explore through a handful of examples and studies.

Unfortunately, their names do not roll off the tongue, but I'll try to share my tricks for remembering their names and functions.

The Cellular Science of Aging: Tricking Our Cells into Scarcity Mode for Longer Life

The current understanding of aging at a cellular level is that there are two modes for cells to be in—the "yin and yang" of cell states, if you will. The yin mode is defense and conservation while the yang mode is growth and reproduction.

Dr. David Sinclair, a foremost longevity researcher, calls the defensive yin mode "hunkering down." Cells hunker down to conserve resources, recycle old parts and stop reproducing —an energy-intensive activity. When resources are abundant and there are no threats, cells go into the growth and reproduction mode, which is counterproductive to longevity. The key to longevity is for the cells to go into the defensive or hunkering-down state which is activated when there is threat or hardship such as inadequate food or other adverse conditions.

For longevity, the optimal trigger is when the threat is mild and stimulates the cells into defense mode but does not represent a mortal challenge. If this mild challenge sounds similar to a hormetic challenge, it is because it is. Remember that too much of a threat to the system (stress, malnutrition) damages your posterior heaven and can shorten your life. So, how do we safely get our cells to switch into hunker-down mode and to switch on our longevity genes?

Toughening up for the Long Haul with Longevity Genes

Dr. Sinclair and other longevity researchers have discovered that there are certain mammalian genes that code for cell switching from growth to defensiveness and are considered longevity genes. In Dr. Sinclair's book *Lifespan: Why We Age— and Why We Don't Have To*, he writes:

> *Together, these genes form a surveillance network within our bodies, communicating with one another between cells and between organs by releasing proteins and chemicals into the bloodstream, monitoring, responding to what we eat, how much we exercise and what time of*

day it is. They tell us to hunker down when the going gets tough and to grow fast and reproduce fast when the going gets easier. [4]

Dr. Sinclair's focus has been on ways to exploit these genes, the first of which are protein enzymes called *sirtuins*.

How Sirtuins Tell the DNA What to Do

Sirtuins change the packaging of DNA, turning genes on and off when needed, which is epigenetics in action. To help me remember how sirtuin proteins function, I imagine them saying to the DNA, "Sir, do it," a mnemonic phrase that sounds like *sir-tu-in*.

Epigenesis, the process by which the instructions in our DNA are converted into a functional product such as a protein, changes how genes are expressed. While epigenesis does not change the DNA itself, sirtuins control which DNA is exposed and expressed, which can maintain our health, fitness and survival. Writer Graham Averill explains the process well:

> *If [our cells] get overwhelmed, [they] start to misbehave, and we see the symptoms of aging, like organ failure or wrinkles. All the genetic info in our cells is still there as we get older, but our body loses the ability to interpret it. This is because our body starts to run low on NAD, a molecule that activates the sirtuins: we have half as much NAD in our body when we're 50 as we do at 20. Without it, the sirtuins can't do their job, and the cells in our body forget what they're supposed to be doing.* [5]

In his own writing, Dr. Sinclair summarizes the reason for aging as a loss of information. We know aging doesn't mean losing the information in DNA, since old cloned cells are as good as young ones. But we *do* lose the ability to accurately access the information on the DNA. This is an example of epigenetics, or how our posterior heaven influences our anterior heaven.

Reduce, Reuse, Recycle: The Roles of TOR and Autophagy

Another important longevity gene is the *target of rapamycin* (TOR or mTOR in mammals), a complex of proteins that regulates growth and metabolism. TOR is sensitive to nutrients, and when it is inhibited and senses nutrients are scarce, it signals cells in stress to go into defensive mode. This way, the cells can improve their chances of survival amid scarcity by boosting such activities as DNA repair and reducing inflammation caused by old and worn cells. But TOR's most crucial function, perhaps, is digesting old, damaged proteins which might otherwise lead to toxic aging.

As mentioned, when TOR is inhibited, it signals scarcity and forces cells to hunker down, making them divide less and forcing them to reuse old cellular components to maintain energy and extend survival. This is a process called *autophagy*, which means "self-eating." I remember the term TOR by imagining the Norse god Thor thrashing around and eating himself when he can't escape his cell (when he is *inhibited*, in other words).

Self-eating, or autophagy, is a function that works to conserve and clean up. Think of it as a mechanic scavenging old auto parts to keep an old car running, as Dr. Sinclair describes, but with the side benefit of cleaning up and organizing the junkyard at the same time. If times are tough, you do not buy a new car; you use whatever you can find to keep going. Similarly, when the going gets tough, shutting down TOR permits cellular survival or longevity and survival of the organism. Therefore, if we are slightly challenged by hunger or other hormetics, our cells see this as a time to conserve and recycle for the long haul, hence leading to longer life.

AMPK: The Metabolic Master Switch

Here's another tongue-twister for you: 5' adenosine monophosphate-activated protein kinase, or more simply, AMPK, is another enzyme that evolved to respond to adverse conditions. AMPK is known as a metabolic master switch when it comes to hunkering down.

AMPK plays a role in cellular energy homeostasis by activating stored glucose and fatty acid uptake when cellular energy is low. Researchers consider AMPK an important therapeutic target for controlling human diseases, including metabolic syndrome and cancer. The type 2 diabetes drug metformin increases AMPK in our cells. AMPK is also affected by curcumin and ginseng, herbs found in Dr. One's medicine bag.

How Defective Insulin-like Growth Factor 1 (IGF-1) Leads to Long Life

You've likely read about (and maybe know) centenarians who confound neighbors, family and researchers. They reach a ripe old age despite a life of eating and drinking whatever they want. In many cases, these centenarians have a gene mutation that codes for faulty insulin-like growth factor 1 (IGF-1). IGF-1 is *reduced* in fasting and fasting-mimicking diets, and these lucky individuals carry gene variants that put their cells in a state of fasting no matter what they eat. This reduction in IGF-1 is associated with lower rates of death and disease, and some researchers have used IGF-1 to predict—with great accuracy—how long someone will live.[6] Those centenarians with an IGF-1 mutation are simply winners in the genetic lottery. They can eat fatty food, drink alcohol and generally be careless with their habits. The rest of us have work to do.

Hormesis: Turning On Our Longevity Genes

Biological stress activates all of these defense systems mentioned above, but some stressors are simply too great to overcome. These stressors cause DNA breaks and mutations leading to illness and death. In Sandra's case, her fear and stress were so overwhelming that it caused her ovaries to start shutting down (stop reproducing), sending her immediately into menopause. But if we use some of Dr. One's hormetic strategies, we may be able to mimic the lucky centenarians I mentioned before. Stressors that activate our longevity genes without damaging the cell are a classic example of hormesis. There are strategies that allow us to expose our bodies to them intentionally to activate our longevity genes.

Lifestyle Strategies for Longevity: Do Not Get Too Comfortable

The lifestyle strategies that help us trick our cells into thinking there is scarcity and to switch into "hunker-down" mode could be summarized as "don't let yourself get too comfortable." Some of these strategies include time-restricted eating, exercise, sauna and cold shock. These tactics must be employed in a hormetic dosage (otherwise, they can be damaging). Let's look at these and others.

Calorie Restriction

Calorie restriction has been shown to prolong life in yeast, fruit flies and mice and anecdotally in humans. As Dr. Sinclair wrote in *Lifespan*, "If this happened only in yeast, it would merely be interesting. But because we knew that rodents also lived longer when their food was restricted it was apparent that this genetic program is very old, perhaps nearly as old as life itself."

In animal studies, the key to engaging the longevity genes is through razor's edge calorie restriction: just enough food to function and no more. This razor's edge is the limiting factor in studying the same effect in humans, since malnutrition can shorten life and is quite unpleasant. A better option is something called intermittent fasting.

Intermittent Fasting

Intermittent fasting is a sustainable caloric restriction strategy. Subjects who followed a restricted diet for five days a month lost weight, reduced their body fat impacting their levels of IGF-1, which as mentioned is a gene linked to longevity.[7] Short of fasting for days each month, a popular strategy is spending 16 hours a day without eating. By eliminating breakfast and having just a small lunch and an early dinner, you can experience some of the benefits of fasting. Almost any periodic fasting diet that does not lead to malnutrition will likely put the longevity genes to work in ways that will result in deep resilience and a longer, healthier life.

Protein Restriction

Limiting your meat and dairy intake reduces protein consumption, inhibiting mTOR and forcing cells to spend less energy dividing and more energy in autophagy. This autophagy leads to the recycling of damaged and misfolded proteins. Recycling: good for the planet and good for your longevity too.

We cannot live without protein, but we can do a better job of restricting the amount we put into our bodies. Part of a good longevity strategy is to cut back on our intake of the amino acid methionine, found in beef, lamb, poultry, pork and eggs, and to substitute it with plant protein.

Exercise

Scientists have found that those adults who exercise more have longer telomeres. People who exercised for the equivalent of at least half an hour of jogging five days a week had telomeres that appeared to be nearly a decade younger than those who lived a more sedentary life. Exercise, by definition, is the application of stress to our bodies, making it a great hormetic strategy for longevity.

The longevity regulators AMPK, mTOR and sirtuins are all modulated in the right direction by exercise, irrespective of caloric intake. They help build new blood vessels, improve heart and lung health, make people stronger and extend telomeres. Even 15 minutes of jogging a day reduced subjects' chance of death from heart attack by 40 percent and all-cause mortality by 45 percent.[8] And 10 minutes a day of high-intensity exercise, the kind that leaves you breathless and sweating, engages the greatest number of health-promoting genes, and more of them in older exercisers.

Cold and Heat

Exposing your body to extreme cold and heat is another effective way to turn on your longevity genes. Cold activates a gene called UCP2, which promotes brown fat in the arms, back and shoulders, leading to more mitochondria (the powerhouses of metabolism). Having enough brown fat can significantly reduce the risk of developing diabetes, obesity and Alzheimer's disease. Exercising in the cold can turbocharge the creation of brown fat, and even sleeping in the cold can help.

The heat of a sauna has beneficial effects too. Researchers studied a group of about 2,300 middle-aged men from Eastern Finland for more than 20 years, and those who used the sauna with great frequency (up to seven times a week) enjoyed a twofold drop in fatal heart attacks. [9] The frequent sauna-goers also had a reduction in all causes of death compared to those who only took one sauna per week. A little stress outside of the thermal neutral zone can go a long way to deepen strength.

Metformin and Rapamycin

Two medications that have received attention in the longevity industry are metformin, the time-honored oral medication for Type 2 diabetes, and rapamycin. A large-scale clinical trial called Targeting Aging by Metformin (TAME) is studying metformin for its positive effects on all-cause mortality independent of its hypoglycemic actions. [10] Metformin regulates mTOR and sirtuins, leading to lower IGF-1 and activating AMPK. The results of the TAME study should offer more guidance on the safety and efficacy of this medication in countering aging.

Rapamycin has been shown to prolong lifespan in flies, yeast and mice through TOR, the receptor that the drug is named for (target of rapamycin). [11] In humans, the downsides to rapamycin therapy include ulcers of mouth and lips, hyperglycemia and diabetes, hyperlipidemia and hypercholesterolemia. These side effects may only be acceptable in conditions with no known cure, such as Alzheimer's disease.

A note of caution: medications can easily tip us into Dr. Three territory with unexpected and undesirable side effects, no matter how convenient a solution may appear. Of course, it is easier to take a pill than jump into the cold bay! Remember: Let other people be the final guinea pigs. We want to follow the Dr. One approach, harnessing the body's own systems with lifestyle changes and acupuncture.

Fruits and Vegetables as a Hormetic Challenge

Another counterintuitive application of the hormetic challenge is the idea that fruits and vegetables may be good for you, not necessarily because of their vitamin or fiber content. Instead, it's the low levels of toxins found in them designed to ward off predators.

My Chinese medicine training taught me that while fruits and vegetables are undoubtedly healthy, the best are grown *near* your home—or better still, *at* your home. We now see that this old folk wisdom may be because the toxins produced by vegetables or fruit grown in your locale are more likely to be effective against actual adverse environments you will encounter.

Fruits and vegetables have innate antifungal, anti-bacterial and anti-grazing properties. The anti-grazing properties might be the tannins in grapes or the spicy nature of some vegetables. But eating these plants, which have developed these aspects of their make-up to survive, makes you tougher too. Though this sounds outlandish, I've become open-minded about old folk wisdom—which brings us to antioxidants.

Are Antioxidants Really Good for Us?

It's widely accepted that antioxidants, substances that protect your cells against free radicals, are vital for good health. Still, an interesting application of the principle of Dr. Three backed up by research shows that antioxidants may do more harm than good—because, in effect, they take away a hormetic challenge.[12] Longevity researcher Dr. Nick Lane points out that antioxidants dampen internal stress response in the cells and weaken them by doing so.[13] His metaphor is that it is like taking away a smoke detector: the smoke and damage remain, but the cell fails to protect itself.

All of these strategies involve effort but are powerful if adopted as habits. Fortunately, we can get many of the same potent anti-aging effects from acupuncture, which also has the advantage of being relaxing and not requiring any effort. Among many other benefits, acupuncture is a type of hormesis since it affects longevity genes. It is no wonder that acupuncture has been highly valued for centuries not only as a treatment for illness, but also for well-being and long life.

Acupuncture as Longevity Hack

Reducing the Stress Response with Acupuncture

There is a real connection between acupuncture and longevity. In fact, research consistently shows that acupuncture improves autonomic balance with increased rest-and-digest activity and decreased fight-or-flight. As we have seen, this improved balance has multiple health advantages. In addition, patients who show improved autonomic balance with acupuncture are much more likely to show clinical improvement over time as well. This measured improvement is a harbinger of better resilience, leading to better results.

Complexity Factors

We know that in addition to giving a snapshot of autonomic function, heart rate variability (HRV) measures the complexity of heart rate response. As we age, we lose complexity across functions ranging from gait to heart rate. Maintaining complexity across different physiological processes can help delay the aging process. Therefore, improving HRV through acupuncture may improve our resilience and longevity.

Other areas of complexity may benefit from acupuncture

as well. For instance, one study showed giving vibrational input to the soles of the feet, or 12 weeks of Tai Chi training analogous to acupuncture treatment, improved balance in elderly patients.[14] This brings us to the topic of acupuncture and how it connects to the ancient concept of *jing*.

Acupuncture and Jing

We have direct evidence that acupuncture in animals can improve physiological measures that are markers of aging. One study showed that acupuncture on the kidney meridian, said to be closely related to *jing*, improved renal function and increased sex hormone production to levels equivalent to that of a younger animal. More research on this type of direct hormonal response is necessary, but the results are provocative.

Acupuncture Provides Cellular Hormesis

Besides harnessing the relaxation response, improving complexity, and increasing hormonal levels, the science of aging shows us other ways acupuncture might help prolong life as a highly effective hormetic challenge. There is now scientific research behind how acupuncture works to improve our longevity through various pathways. We'll start with AMPK.

AMPK

Some animal studies show that electro acupuncture activates the AMPK system.[15] Remember, AMPK is activated by the drug Metformin, now the subject of the TAME trial. If we can activate that same system with acupuncture reliably, it would be safer, since acupuncture triggers the body's own cascades, so there are minimal side effects. Dr. One wants to do no harm, and though metformin may be helpful, using acupuncture to do the same thing keeps the system balanced and less likely to spiral out of control. While these studies ask more questions than they answer, they are nonetheless encouraging and help to provide insight into the prevention and anti-aging aspect of ancient acupuncture treatments.

Sirtuins

Additional studies have shown that acupuncture affects sirtuins. As noted, sirtuins are the "Sir, do it" messengers which help determine which genes will be expressed. In the first study, the authors hypothesize that acupuncture exerts its beneficial effects through epigenesis, improving posterior heaven by way of Sirt2, one of the seven different sirtuins.[16] The second study concerns Sirt1, a sirtuin long recognized for its role in longevity. In this study, they explored its role in mitigating obesity.[17]

Again, these studies were done with animals but may help to guide further acupuncture research. They also bolster the strategy of Dr. One in using acupuncture to help in achieving a long health span.

The mTOR Pathway

Perhaps the most promising studies concern mTOR signaling, showing that mTOR was beneficial in mice with Parkinson's by clearing proteins through the mTOR pathway.[18] Both rapamycin and acupuncture achieved this, but acupuncture did not have any side effects. Similarly, mice with premature ovarian failure averted it through the mTOR pathway as well.[19] It turns out that mTOR may account for the effectiveness of electroacupuncture in patients undergoing in vitro fertilization (IVF).[20] Acupuncture likely acts as a longevity hormetic stimulus by activating the "hunkering-down" switch of mTOR—which leads to the discussion of how herbal therapy can aid in longevity as a radical prevention strategy.

Herbal Therapy: Astragalus

Herbal therapy is an integral part of Chinese medicine, though I haven't stressed it here because it would require a book of its own. But to broaden our mental models, I will share a little about astragalus, an herb used in formulas to boost immunity and longevity.[21]

Astragalus can be taken daily, usually with other herbs, for prevention. In Chinese medicine, these types of formulas are called tonics and are part of the overall radical prevention strategy, used to fortify your system. Researchers have studied this popular herb and found that astragalus lengthens telomeres.[22] Injected astragalus also increases autophagy, cleaning up senescent proteins and cells through the AMPK-mTOR pathway, and decreases IL-6, a pro-inflammatory protein.[23]

Wildcards and the Profound Effects of Posterior Heaven/Epigenetics

With a better grasp of the science explaining how acupuncture affects the body, we now have a greater understanding of the significance of Sandra's story. Her circumstances took her into the center of a violent encounter between two dogs, and the severe fright and stress to her system damaged "her kidneys," according to Chinese medicine. As a result, her fertility started to decline toward menopause. We can now widen our mental models to allow for how acupuncture might have allowed her to maintain her fertility and then conceive. But perhaps above all, her story illustrates the profound effects epigenesis, or our posterior heaven, can have on our lives—particularly when life throws us dangerous wildcards. Longevity is starting to be recognized as a valid aim in modern medicine, though modern medicine is late to the party, of course, compared to Chinese medicine. By looking at the science as we currently know it, it seems that by promoting stress reduction and hormetic challenges through acupuncture and lifestyle changes, we can build some of the radical resilience required to reach 100 years and beyond.

Chapter 5
Our Immune System: Defender and Slayer

"Like police in a time of martial law, the immune system seeks out threats and keeps them from doing mortal harm, ably discerning up to a billion different alien hazards, even ones not yet discovered by science."
–Matt Richtel, *An Elegant Defense*

When Christopher Lynn, PhD, an associate professor of anthropology at the University of Alabama, got himself a tattoo, the process physically drained him. "They don't just hurt while you get the tattoo, but they can exhaust you," he said. "It's easier to get sick. You can catch a cold because your defenses are lowered from the stress of getting a tattoo."[1]

Inspired by his personal experience, Lynn published a study in the *American Journal of Human Biology* called "Tattooing to 'Toughen Up': Tattoo experience and secretory Immunoglobulin A."[2] The study found that levels of immunoglobulin A dropped significantly in those getting a tattoo for the first time, weakening the immune system and causing an upper respiratory tract infection. Significantly, the immunoglobulin A decrease was less marked among those who received tattoos more frequently; repeated over time, tattoos decreased the effect. Dr. Lynn summed it up like so:

"When receiving a tattoo, the body mobilizes immunological agents to fight possible infections at the site of the new tattoo. Repeated tattooing makes your immune system stronger."

So, what can tattoos teach us about the immune system and how to make it stronger? As Dr. Lynn's research helps illustrate, the body's response to tattooing is akin to exercising when you're out of shape. Initially, the muscles become sore— but if you continue, the soreness fades, and after subsequent workouts, the muscles become stronger (an example of hormesis, a favorite tool of Dr. One). While this counterintuitive research did not at all surprise acupuncturists, it would be understandable for many to discount it as an outlier or a mistake, or to argue that "correlation is not causation." Even so, the argument makes much more sense if we look closer at the immune system, which we will do in this chapter.

Understanding the intricacies of the immune system will help us explain the alarming rise in autoimmune diseases, which occur when the immune system mistakenly attacks the body's own healthy tissues; on the other end of the spectrum, we'll uncover the body's devastating lack of an immune response to cancer, a phenomenon that has confounded scientists for decades. We will learn the surprising truth that it's possible to be "too clean" and the paradoxical consequences of our increasingly sterile modern lifestyles. In a journey to Sardinia, we'll learn how the absence of certain beneficial parasites can lead to autoimmune diseases. We will also travel to Mexico where we will meet a gonzo journalist who travels there to infect himself with a parasitic worm in his quest to quell his own autoimmune condition. And we will see how research has shown that the detailed mechanisms from nerve endings to brain and back again sheds light on how acupuncture can regulate the immune response with profound effects.

Before we continue, it's important to appreciate that the immune system is involved with debilitating and life-threatening conditions such as cancer, Alzheimer's, diabetes, COVID-19, flu, stress, pain and stroke. It involves mind-bending biochemistry, the autonomic nervous system (which controls unconscious bodily functions such as breathing, heartbeat and digestion) and the stress response. It's also important to understand that the immune system works as a feedback system maintaining homeostasis.

Immune Dysfunction in Public Health: Scope of the Problem

Immune dysfunction is at the root of many common illnesses, even the big killers like cancer and heart disease. Not only do we need to mount a healthy response to invading microbes or other interlopers (splinters, poisons), but we also do not want our bodies to overdo it, leading to autoimmune conditions. As Matt Richtel, author of *An Elegant Defense: The Extraordinary New Science of the Immune System*, writes, "An unchecked immune system can grow so zealous that it turns as dangerous as any foreign disease."[3]

We need to keep our immune system balanced so that it defends us without overdoing it. To understand how important this is, note that the immune system is so powerful that the body makes certain areas off-limits to it, such as the brain and the eyes. As we will see, the autonomic nervous system plays a crucial role in keeping the immune system from overheating and attacking our own tissues.

Autoimmunity is on the rise, affecting 20 percent of Americans—some 50 million people. It is the third most common disease, while diabetes, the seventh leading killer, is caused by the immune system going to war against the pancreas. Moises Velasquez-Manoff, author of *An Epidemic of Absence: A New Way of Understanding Allergies and Autoimmune Diseases*, colorfully imagines the widespread impact of immune dysfunction if he had superhuman power to see everything happening in the world around him. He writes:

> *Walking down Broadway in New York City, for instance, one of every ten children passing by would have asthma; one in six would have an itchy rash and sometimes blisters—eczema. One of every five passersby would have hay fever. If I could see allergic antibodies directly—immunoglobulin—I'd note that half the crowd around me was sensitized to dust mites, tree pollen, and peanuts, among other basically harmless proteins. I'd see pockets full of inhalers, and bags stuffed with allergy medicines. In the satchels of the most severely afflicted, I'd see pills of powerful immune suppressants, such as prednisone. I'd even see a few soon to be corpses; about 3,500 people die yearly from asthma attacks.*[4]

The financial cost of autoimmunity is also high. For example, the direct and indirect costs of asthma combined reach about $56 billion a year. With this and other autoimmune diseases, funds flow to doctors and drug companies while workers take sick days and overall productivity is diminished.

If we could tame our out-of-control immune systems, it would save money and radically improve people's lives. Of course, too little immune response can result in cancer. As Richtel writes in his book, "Cancer can play a nasty trick on this elegant defense [of our immune system]. Cancer can tell [it] to 'stand down.' It then uses the immune system to protect the cancer."[5] With all this in mind, was Dr. Lynn onto something with his observations about tattoos? Was he perhaps giving us a peek into the workings of Dr. One?

What Is the Immune System?

Recognizing Friend from Foe

The immune system is one of our bodies' most sophisticated and extensive feedback loops with the heroic task of detecting and attacking invaders and welcoming foreign substances such as food and beneficial bacteria. The surveillance of the immune system and its various squadrons of cells and messengers that live in the skin, tissues, lymph organs and plasma are discerning and extremely powerful.

Our vital microbiome (the community of microorganisms in our body) consists of both helpful and harmful microbes that reside in our skin, mouth, nose and GI tract. In total, this makes up about four pounds of bacteria, some of which are essential to our survival and must be welcomed and not eradicated. Our immune systems must be able to identify the helpful ones and limit the harmful ones—quite a task! It is a testament to the immune system's success that we are still alive at all.

The classic medical textbook *Cellular and Molecular Immunology* by Abul K. Abbas, Andrew H. Lichtman and Shiv Pillai states immune principles best: "Every individual's immune system is able to recognize, respond to and eliminate many foreign (non-self) antigens but does not usually react against that individual's own (self) antigens and tissues. Different mechanisms are used by the innate and adaptive immune systems to prevent reactions against healthy self-cells."[6]

This means that antigens, which are markers on foreign substances and our own tissues, are how the immune system recognizes friend from foe. With spectacular accuracy, the immune system recognizes these markers almost like keys in a lock, keeping out invaders and leaving our own tissues, food and friendly bacteria alone.

Lymphocytes and other immune cells can circulate among tissues, meaning immunity is a systemic phenomenon. An immune response initiated in one part of the body can protect other parts of the body, a feature that is essential for the success of vaccination. A vaccine administered in the subcutaneous or muscle tissue of the arm can protect us from infections in *any* tissue.

Immune responses are regulated by feedback loops that amplify the reaction and control mechanisms that prevent inappropriate or disease-related reactions. When lymphocytes are activated, they trigger mechanisms that further increase the magnitude of the response. This is the most important positive feedback that enables the small number of lymphocytes specific for any microbe to generate a large response to eradicate that infection. In addition, negative feedback mechanisms become active during immune responses. These prevent excessive activation of lymphocytes against "self-antigens" that could cause collateral damage to normal tissues.

Through all these details, it's important to reiterate the bigger point: the immune system uses both positive *and* negative feedback systems to keep itself running smoothly. As Matt Richtel writes in *An Elegant Defense*, "The story of the immune system became the story of homeostasis—a state of harmony or stability. It is a system precisely and delicately tailored to stay in balance."[7] He further illustrates this point with some history, specifically a story about Russian zoologist Elie Metchnikoff.

Elie Metchnikoff and the Beginnings of Immunology

In the summer of 1882, Russian zoologist Elie Metchnikoff, troubled by intensifying persecution of Jewish farmers, left his homeland to stay with his sister on the Mediterranean island of Sicily. Metchnikoff was studying starfish larvae, and because they are transparent, he could easily observe their cell workings through a microscope. He dubbed the cells he saw moving through these tiny organisms "wandering cells" and wondered if they might serve in defense of the starfish larvae. In search of an answer, he put rose thorns from his sister's garden under the skin of the larvae. Would the cells somehow swarm and protect?

The following day, after a sleepless night of anticipation, he peered through his microscope and experienced the classic "aha" moment—"The great event of my scientific life," he wrote. The wandering cells swarmed around the splinter, eating away at it and the damaged tissues. With this simple experiment, Metchnikoff developed the "phagocyte" theory— phagocytosis means "cell eating," a process of defense against invaders and a way to clean up damaged tissues.

Subsequently, he connected this phenomenon to immune defense in humans, in which pus forms in response to a splinter or injury and generalized inflammation occurs through injury. Describing inflammation, Metchnikoff said, "At the moment of invasion, the body has an initial reaction that involves the swarming of eater cells, and the experience is not always pleasant." Metchnikoff's brilliant hunch led to a major discovery that launched the science and discipline of immunology.

Aspects of the Immune System

Innate Immune System: The Body's Standing Army for Emergency Reaction

The skin is our immune system's first line of defense, as the integrity of our skin repels many invaders by providing a protective barrier. Our version of the starfish larvae's wandering cells—neutrophils and macrophages—are a standing army that lives in the tissues and cells throughout our bodies, ready to charge into action in the presence of an invader. This is our innate immune system, and it usually defends against microbes by invoking inflammation, but sometimes without it.

These equivalents to wandering cells also sound the alarm and send chemical messengers that cause dilation of the blood vessels near the injury, creating an offramp so neutrophils (the most abundant type of white blood cells) can assemble. These reactions lead to inflammation (redness, heat, swelling and pain) and neutrophils or pus.

The skin has an ever-present army of sentinel phagocytic cells and nerve endings ready to react to invaders. In response to injury and inflammation, pain receptors transmit signals to the brain stem which then sends a message *through the vagus nerve* to limit inflammation. Without this signaling and homeostasis, the body would overreact and spiral out of control. Remember: we saw in Chapter 3 that acupuncture blunted the autonomic response to startle in beagles and horses.

If the immune system is not kept in check, various autoimmune diseases such as rheumatoid arthritis and allergic rhinitis can arise, as well as sepsis and the "cytokine storm" associated with COVID-19. This helps explain how the slight "injury" invoked by the needles in tattooing and acupuncture can trigger a healing response through vagal stimulation or an increase in rest-and-digest activity. As Abbas and colleagues state in their textbook *Cellular and Molecular Immunology*, "The innate immune response to microbes provides early danger signals that stimulate the adaptive immune system."[8] To explain what this means, let's take a closer look at adaptive immunity.

Adaptive Immunity: The Immune System's Long-Term Memory

Adaptive immunity, also called specific immunity or acquired immunity, leverages the highly intricate mechanisms in the body in which we mount a specific reaction to a toxin, bacteria or virus invader. This process involves a series of messengers that stimulate B cells to clone themselves and make antibodies specific to that invader. While this takes six to seven days, it can be devastatingly effective. Introducing a small amount of a toxin or a portion of a virus to the body, by way of a vaccine, enables it to respond and then *have a memory* of that invader to halt future attacks.

The concept is not new—the ancient Chinese made children resistant to smallpox by having them breathe powders from the skin lesions of patients recovering from the disease, a primitive but effective means of invoking the immune system. And in the late 1700s, British physician Edward Jenner pioneered vaccines by famously inoculating people with material from cowpox sores which conferred immunity to human smallpox.

The tricky part of vaccines is to give the immune system a small enough piece of the virus so that it does not infect us, but enough that it will stimulate an immune response if we are confronted with the virus again. If the invader attacks, even years later, the memory of it is present, and our bodies quickly clone antibodies and launch a defense. The immune system can then distinguish friend from foe, destroying substances that contain the virus' offending antigens as quickly as the virus can replicate. This helps explain the rationale behind giving plasma from people who have successfully recovered from COVID-19 to others with severe infections: it can supply a temporary boost in immunoglobulins to lower the numbers of invaders until the patient's immune system takes over during the six to seven days needed to clone the antibodies.

Our powerful immune system can immediately detect and attack incoming foes and has the mind-blowing ability to memorize everything it encounters. It is so fantastic it seems like science fiction, but it isn't. It's the genius of our physiology, our own "elegant defense." But the immune system has the power to hurt us, too. It is not perfect.

To help our immune system, the mental model that has to bend is that we don't want to be "too clean." We must acknowledge that our ancient "old friends" of bacteria and parasites can be sorely missed once they are gone, leaving a propensity for allergy and autoimmunity in their wake. To illustrate this, we'll follow the journey of a fearless journalist who tried to reintroduce worms to his system.

The Immune System's Lost "Old Friends" and the Hygiene Hypothesis

How do we toughen up and keep resilient? There's a concept in immunology called "old friends," or the evolutionary theory, and its counterpart, the hygiene hypothesis. In this concept, bacteria and parasites were our constant companions since humankind began. Without them, as the theory goes in immunology, our immune systems can flounder and potentially even turn against us.

Dr. Meg Lemon, a prominent dermatologist, internist and expert in autoimmune disease, paints a vivid (and only slightly facetious) picture of this idea:

> *I tell people, when they drop food on the floor, please pick it up and eat it. Get rid of the antibacterial soap. Immunize! We have animals in our homes, and they sleep with us. If your dog shits on the floor, clean it up, of course, but don't use bleach. You should not only pick your nose, you should eat it. Our immune system needs a job. We evolved over millions of years to have our immune systems under constant assault. Now they don't have anything to do.*[9]

The hygiene hypothesis refers to the counterintuitive conundrum that if we are too clean, we can suffer unintended consequences like allergies. When the term was first coined in Britain in the 1800s to describe hay fever, an allergy was seen as an affliction of the upper, monied classes. As it turned out, allergies were a function of the lack of "old friends." Allergies only afflicted those whose living conditions and environment were clean enough to avoid exposure to animal dander and dirt.

Our immune systems evolved over millennia while exposed to animal dander and dirt, which primed the immune system to fight. When we take them away, there is nothing for the immune system to do, so it overreacts to harmless challenges. It is still the case that allergies and autoimmune diseases are not as frequent in the less hygienic developing world. In the absence of dirt and dander in the Western world, our bodies overreact to false foes, like pollen, nuts or grasses. To illustrate this point, we can look at a sobering public health trend in northern Sardinia.

Sardinia, Multiple Sclerosis and the Lack of Old Foes

Northern Sardinia is sometimes considered a playground for the wealthy, brimming with expensive yachts and blessed with isolated beaches. Away from the pristine beaches are ancient structures called *nuraghe*, a word from the native language spoken before the Romans arrived 2,000 years ago.

During that time, *nuraghe*, which roughly translates to "a pile of stones," were already 1,500 years old. Primitive but sturdy, hollow inside and shaped slightly like medieval towers, approximately 7,000 remain on the island today. Ancient Sardinians may have built them as status symbols or lookouts, but there's also a theory that the *nuraghe* provided an escape from the ever-present mosquito, which brought malaria, meaning "bad air," to the island. In Cagliari, the island's capital, there is even a Roman Catholic shrine for the Virgin Mary called The Basilica of Our Lady of *Bonaria*, or "good air."

Since inhabitants of Sardinia are historically isolated island dwellers, they have a concentrated genetic imprint. While their genetics protect against malaria, that same code can increase autoimmune disease. Sixty years ago, malaria was common; while many succumbed to it, many survived, seemingly resistant to the parasite. After the eradication of malaria in the 1950s, autoimmune diseases like multiple sclerosis and type 1 diabetes skyrocketed. Sardinians now have one of the highest levels of autoimmune disease in the world and are two to three times more likely to develop multiple sclerosis than residents of neighboring islands or mainland Italians.[10]

The theory is that the Sardinians' immune systems evolved to battle the malaria parasite. Over time, they *needed* to battle it, otherwise their immune systems would attack their own tissues, tipping into autoimmunity. In other words, the genes that protected the population against the "old friend" malaria turned inward on the population after the malaria eradication. The Sardinia story is one of the most dramatic examples of how our immune systems evolved over millennia, and how they cannot suddenly (well, within a generation or two) adapt to a new reality.

Author Moises Velasquez-Manoff describes a similar phenomenon related to parasites in *An Epidemic of Absence*, detailing a personal journey of discovery motivated by severe allergies and an autoimmune condition.

Remove Worms and Allergies Flourish

In his book *An Epidemic of Absence*, author Velasquez-Manoff explains the concepts behind "old friends" and how autoimmune diseases are more common where parasites have been eliminated. It also details his personal journey of discovery, motivated by severe allergies and an autoimmune condition that caused him to lose all his body hair before the age of 18.

He learned of anecdotal evidence that reintroducing hookworm could trick a person's immune system into standing down and not attacking itself, calming down autoimmune disease and leaving the hair follicles, skin and lungs alone. Eventually, he took the radical step of traveling to Mexico to purchase and self-inoculate with hookworm, an "old friend" capable of disabling our immune systems so that it might coexist with us in our gastrointestinal tracts. His book outlines the incredible science behind our complicated relationship with parasites, dirt and bacteria. One aspect of his experience caught my attention and warrants emphasis: the phenomenon called "hookworm high."

Hookworm High

Velasquez-Manoff reported that one patient inoculated with hookworm said his skin "seemed a little less angry almost immediately." And that an odd feeling of euphoria overtook him on the flight home, saying that he "wanted to get up and do cartwheels." Velasquez-Manoff wondered if this "hook-worm high" could relate to a cessation of inflammation-mediated depression, something that others who self-inoculated reported to have experienced.[11] And it is also possible that this feeling results from the vagal aspect of the autonomic nervous system.

The triggering of healing from acupuncture provokes the rest-and-digest aspect of the autonomic nervous system, commonly leading to feelings of well-being. This can be a feeling of relaxation or heaviness, or sometimes bliss and euphoria. This feeling could indicate the triggering of the vagus nerve in response to needling and account for the improvement in immunity with tattoos. The use of hookworm to treat autoimmune disease remains more theoretical than efficacious, but it has served as fodder for new approaches to the widespread and pernicious problem of autoimmunity.

Of course, most people won't infect themselves with worms or get a tattoo, so what else can we do? As it turns out, acupuncture can help prime the immune system, too.

The Science of Acupuncture and Immunity: Getting Under Your Skin

The response to the introduction of an acupuncture needle into the skin is like that observed by Metchnikoff when starfish larvae mounted a cellular reaction to that rose thorn. A significant difference, however, is that the skin is part of a complex web of cascading reactions involving adjacent tissues, the bloodstream and lymphoid tissues.

A splinter in the skin stimulates white blood cells to the region and local phagocytosis (cell eating, as discussed earlier). Acupuncture, for the most part, stimulates processes in this innate immune system. Though it is non-specific, it still stimulates feedback mechanisms that can be useful to keep the immune system in balance.

Meet the Neuroendocrine Immune Response

The term neuroendocrine immune response might sound intimidating, but it simply refers to the signals the skin transmits by nerves, hormonal systems and the immune system. As discussed, the skin reacts to injury just like the starfish larvae, but nerves signal the brain stem which, in turn, sends messages through the vagus nerve to limit inflammation. The sentinel cells communicate with circulating cells to dilate the blood vessels so that neutrophils can swarm the area. If this reaction is not kept in check—as with severe COVID-19, for example—we see havoc wrought by severe clotting and inflammation of the lungs. Sepsis is another example of the body's often lethal overreaction to a bacterial infection.

The minor "injury" evoked by needles can trigger a healing response. When done a few times, as in tattooing, it keeps the immune system steady but alert. This evolutionary response to an injury keeps the body from spiraling out of control, as Dr. One intuitively understood.

Acupuncture Stimulates Processes in the Innate Immune System

Researchers at China's Tianjin University of Traditional Chinese Medicine found that acupuncture needles could cause the muscle fibers to fracture in the acupuncture points after needle insertion, with many red blood cells and fracture fragments and infiltration of inflammatory cells.[12] If this sounds familiar, it is because this immune reaction to the needle describes the response to any physical invader that breaches the skin. These changes lead to local inflammation in acupuncture points.

In a comprehensive review of acupuncture's effect on the immune system, Sandra Silverio Lopes identifies many immunomodulatory effects of needling.[13] Among them are the mobilization of corticosterone and endorphins, as well as pro-inflammatory and anti-inflammatory effects. Acupuncture and electroacupuncture increased immunity in people with low immunity defenses like cancer patients and the elderly.

Is it "too good to be true" that acupuncture can decrease what needs decreasing and increase what needs increasing? No. Dr. One's method employs techniques that nudge the systems back into homeostasis. With acupuncture, and through the neuroendocrine-immune feedback system which goes up to the brainstem and feeds back to the cellular level through the vagus nerve, the system is either kept in balance or nudged back in balance.

Acupuncture and Adaptive Immunity

Processes related to adaptive immunity, such as the release of natural killer cells (NK cells), are affected by acupuncture. Although NK cells are part of the innate immune response and not the adaptive response, this class of lymphocytes still trigger an adaptive response through the production of interferon (IFN).

Does Acupuncture Work against Allergies?

In an Australian study, acupuncture decreased immunoglobulin (IgE) linked to allergies to dust mites and suppressed the pro-inflammatory neuropeptide substance P.[14] The researchers split 151 individuals into real and sham acupuncture groups. Both groups received twice-weekly treatments for eight weeks; there was also a third "no acupuncture" control group. At the end of the study, only the real acupuncture group experienced significant benefits.

The researchers commented, "Nasal obstruction, nasal itch, sneezing, runny nose, eye itch, and unrefreshed sleep improved significantly in the real acupuncture group (postnasal drip and sinus pain did not) and continued to improve up to four-week follow-up."

Systems Synergy and "Spinning It All Together" through Improved Vagal Tone

Peer-reviewed South Korean research published in *Frontiers in Neuroscience*, a leading journal, showed that patients who responded to acupuncture with less itch in response to histamine also improved their vagal or parasympathetic tone.[15] This research seems to validate my own uncontrolled observational study suggesting that acupuncture responders show pronounced, demonstrable stress reduction in contrast to acupuncture non-responders. [16]

I am not suggesting that simple acupuncture is the ultimate answer to rheumatoid arthritis, multiple sclerosis or even asthma. But given that it has a safe risk/benefit ratio and many explicit mechanisms, this response is likely more than just a placebo, and the Australian study shows it might be a potent immune regulator. If we can study and hone the treatment to evoke more of the regulatory immune response, it could be part of our medicine of the future and our radical resilience and prevention moonshot.

Chapter 6
Inflammation: Silent, Pervasive and Deadly

"If you don't think your anxiety, depression, sadness and stress impact your physical health, think again. All of these emotions trigger chemical reactions in your body, which can lead to inflammation and a weakened immune system. Learn how to cope, sweet friend. There will always be dark days."
—Kris Carr

BD's Story

A patient of mine, BD, is a high-powered financial consultant in her forties. She works for a major company and handles famous, sky-high net worth clients. She is what I call Windex® clean, as she doesn't drink alcohol or coffee, exercises regularly (good posterior heaven) and looks half her age (probably good anterior and posterior heaven). Nonetheless, she has had lifelong issues with constipation, and for a long time only had once-a-week "regularity." Travel, dietary disruption, long workdays and deadlines contributed to the problem. The diagnosis: irritable bowel disease.

BD was referred to me by another patient, and because of her disciplined lifestyle, she kept her weekly appointments.

During treatment, I focused on traditional points for digestion, emphasizing those which have a particular effect on increasing parasympathetic activity and bowel motility. Within a month of sessions, BD's condition improved dramatically, and her regularity went from weekly to daily. Today, BD continues her treatment—at least monthly or as often as her work schedule allows—and has maintained her daily regularity. But how is this possible? How can inserting a few needles into the body dramatically affect a system as complicated as the gut? The evidence presented in this chapter provides clues.

Though inflammation is one of our valuable mechanisms of self-defense, it can spiral out of control without our even knowing it. Inflammation can be "silent," and undetected with deadly consequences. In the last chapter, we became acquainted with some of the immune system's potent feed-back loops. One of the most crucial feedback loops is your rest-and-digest response, which harnesses the vagus nerve and keeps inflammation in check. Because inflammation and its measurement with blood biomarkers and heart rate variability (HRV) are tightly correlated, we can use them to start to detect and treat out-of-control inflammation.

In this chapter, we will meet the innovative researchers using surgically implanted vagal stimulators to battle some of the most aggressive forms of inflammation. I'll reveal the secrets of one of the most commonly used acupuncture points since the ancient times of Dr. One, connecting it to recent pioneering science that shows its power to affect vagal activity. Finally, we will revisit the concept of "old friends" and the paradox of being "too clean" in a fascinating study comparing the stress reactions of city dwellers and farm dwellers, all to give us a better understanding of why some scientists think inflammation underlies most large and small medical conditions.

Inflammation: The Scope of the Problem

Though inflammation is a part of the immune system, it has such enormous effects on health and well-being that it has gained a high profile in modern medicine. Ongoing inflammation in the body can be detrimental to health and mood, ultimately shortening our lifespan. Research shows that factors like obesity, smoking and a sedentary lifestyle partly intensify inflammation, and that inflammation contributes to some of the most challenging and deadly diseases of our time including rheumatoid arthritis, cancer, heart disease, diabetes and asthma. Inflammation can also have an insidious role in mental health, leading to depression, Alzheimer's disease and autism spectrum disorder.

Inflammation is even implicated in longevity—so much so that researchers have coined the term "inflammaging" to describe its effects. As we age, we lose our ability to bring down our inflammation. This increase in inflammation causes an acceleration in the aging process, which leads to even less ability to control the inflammation. This relationship exemplifies a vicious negative feed-forward cycle, one that Dr. One's teachings strive to interrupt. Dr. One would choose to use acupuncture techniques and other means to calm the autonomic nervous system down, preemptively bringing down inflammation and optimizing the body's balance.

Researchers can now measure inflammation precisely in blood markers such as C-reactive protein (CRP), interleukin 6 (IL-6), interleukin 1-B(Il-1β), and Tumor Necrosis Factor (TNF). This specificity helps us to better understand the underlying processes contributing to inflammation and how we can control it. We will see, through the language of modern science, how acupuncture and other strategies stimulate the body's homeostatic feedback systems to decrease both acute and chronic inflammation. Let's look first at acute inflammation.

Acute Inflammation: Four Signs from the Greeks

As far back as the 1st century AD, the ancient Greek philosopher Celsus described the symptoms of inflammation as *rubor*, *calor*, *tumor* and *dolor* (redness, heat, swelling and pain). Acute inflammation is an essential survival mechanism triggered in response to any intruder that breaches the body's integrity. The intruder could be a virus, bacteria, splinter or acupuncture needle. When a breach happens, not all of the hallmarks of inflammation are necessarily present, but a reaction occurs. One of the main characters in this life-and-death struggle are macrophages, a type of immune cell that is constantly looking for injury and foreign invaders.

Macrophages sense and respond to pathogens and other environmental challenges and participate in tissue repair after injury, but most relevant to our discussion is their release of inflammation-inducing *cytokines*. Macrophages release inflammatory messenger cytokines such as tumor necrosis factor (TNF), interleukin 6 (Il-6) and interleukin 1-β (Il1-β) when they encounter intruders.

Cytokines are messengers that can be helpers or destroyers. They cause blood vessels to leak fluid into the tissues, producing swelling (*tumor*), which helps isolate the foreign substance from further contact with body tissues. The cytokines also attract white blood cells called phagocytes that "eat" germs and dead or damaged cells. Redness (*rubor*) occurs because of increased blood flow to these regions, which makes the area warm (*calor*). Pain (*dolor*) occurs because the cytokines aggravate pain receptors.

When Inflammation Is "Too Much of a Good Thing"

Acute inflammation strikes rapidly, usually within minutes, but doesn't last long. This response returns the affected area to a state of balance, inflammation dissipates within a few hours or days, and we then go on our merry way. For this to work correctly, homeostatic feedback systems come into play: our bodies require just enough immune response in the acute situation to combat the intruder, but not too much. Taken to the extreme, a "too much" reaction can culminate in death, with the immune system attacking the body's own tissues in conditions such as sepsis and severe COVID-19. In these situations, the body goes into a death spiral, the ultimate example of spinning out of control.

The serious and life-threatening condition of sepsis is often in response to a bacterial or viral infection. Patients require the highest level of intervention and are usually in the intensive care unit. They can endure damaged lungs, kidneys and other organs and sometimes even die. In the context of COVID-19, a similar negative spiral happens. You may have heard the term "cytokine storm." Benjamin tenOever, an expert in viruses at New York's Icahn School of Medicine, argued in the journal *Cell* that an exaggerated immune response leads to severe COVID-19, which can sometimes cause blood clots, strange swelling in children and ultra-inflammatory cytokine storms.[1] These phenomena have the characteristics of autoimmune disorders in that the immune system attacks tissues in the body instead of actual "foes." *New Yorker* writer James Somers explains it:

> *As the virus spreads unchecked through the body, it drags a destructive immune reaction behind it. Individuals with COVID-19 face the same challenge as nations during the pandemic: if they can't contain small sites of infection early—so that a targeted response can root them out— they end up mounting interventions so large that the shock inflicts its own damage.*[2]

It would be cavalier to say that acupuncture has any significant role in combating these awful, extreme instances of acute inflammation (though there are animal studies that offer evidence to the contrary, which we will explore further on). For the most part, once sepsis or florid COVID-19 take root, we need all the Dr. Twos we can find and should unhesitatingly welcome the miracles of modern medicine. But there are many stealth destabilizing effects of low-grade *chronic* inflammation that Dr. One's laws might reduce.

Chronic Inflammation: A Smoldering Menace

Inflammation is subject to the law of balance, just like all the other conditions discussed in this book. Sometimes, there is ongoing inflammation below the surface. Imagine that the initial inflammation was a wildfire that was mostly put out, but some of its embers are still hidden and burning. These embers are walled off, constantly releasing smoke or inflammatory substances. Because the body cannot find the hidden inflammation, it can't heal itself, and the inflammation becomes chronic.

This chronic inflammation can affect your longevity, mood, immune system and pain. Inflammation is also reflected in your autonomic balance. Heart rate variability (HRV), the complexity measure that reflects the subtle balance of the autonomic nervous system, is highly correlated with the level of inflammation in the body.[3] The higher the inflammation, the unhealthier the HRV.

While sepsis and serious COVID are two examples of acute inflammation getting out of control, most of us are likely more familiar with two common chronic inflammatory conditions: rheumatoid arthritis and inflammatory bowel disease.

Rheumatoid Arthritis

Rheumatoid arthritis is an inflammatory autoimmune condition characterized by flare-ups of swollen, painful, warm and red joints. But rheumatoid arthritis patients also have an ongoing inflammatory process apart from acute flare-ups with heightened inflammatory markers. Since their inflammation is not limited to their joints, they are also more likely to have a shortened lifespan due to heart attacks and cancer.

Inflammatory Bowel Disease

Another common chronic inflammatory condition is inflammatory bowel disease, where the constant inflammation of the gastrointestinal tract causes gastrointestinal distress, constipation and other uncomfortable and sometimes serious ailments. My patient, BD, suffered from this condition; though not disabling, it was still distressing for her.

With chronic inflammation, the "smoldering embers" of ongoing, unabated and hidden inflammation keep the body out of balance. The ancients had no concept of inflammation, no vocabulary for it—but the principles of balance, prevention and hormesis can all be applied to the problems caused by inflammation.

Do No Harm: The First Law of Dr. One and Anti-inflammatory Medications

To truly "do no harm," doctors need to carefully evaluate the risk/benefit of anti-inflammatory medications when advising patients, especially because their systemic effects can often be taken too lightly.

One of the most popular and well-known anti-inflammatory medications is aspirin, which has been used since the 1890s as an anti-inflammatory and antipyretic (fever-lowering) medication. Other long-trusted over-the-counter anti-inflammatory medications have been around for decades as well, such as ibuprofen or naproxen. But while quite effective and safe if used for a few days, they can be brutal to the gastrointestinal tract. In fact, gastroenterologists say that orthopedic surgeons and rheumatologists keep them in business because of the havoc created by anti-inflammatory medications.

We also now have biologics, or monoclonal antibodies, as an anti-inflammatory treatment, which can be highly effective but are limited to certain illnesses. There are also corticosteroids, such as prednisone, which have potent anti-inflammatory action but severe side effects if taken for extended periods.

All these medications have their dangers. Even a baby aspirin a day has been proven to increase bleeding risk, so it is only recommended for people with a known risk of heart attack and stroke. NSAIDs (nonsteroidal anti-inflammatories such as ibuprofen) and even steroids can be safe and beneficial for acute inflammation, but they can destabilize the system when taken for extended periods.

Hormesis: The Second Law of Dr. One and Coaxing the Flywheel

When the body senses an intruder—whether it's a bee sting, cut or another injury—nerves signal the brain and macrophages release cytokine messengers. The brain triggers the hypothalamic-pituitary-adrenal axis, the body's source of cortisol, to dampen inflammation. But it also reacts through the two branches of the autonomic nervous system, providing negative feedback to keep inflammation from spiraling out of control. As we see in COVID-19, the inflammatory cytokine release can be so extreme that it damages the person's own tissues. The autonomic reflex is like *putting the brakes* on this out-of-control inflammatory reaction.

The sympathetic (fight-or-flight) nervous system *decreases* the release of cytokines that lead to more inflammation (Tumor Necrosis Factor-TNF, Il-1B or IL 6) and *increases* those that decrease inflammation (IL-10). But laboratory and clinical evidence shows that the *parasympathetic* nervous system (rest-and-digest) plays the leading role in reducing inflammation. This vagal, parasympathetic rest-and-digest outflow affects the major organ systems and tissue macrophages (surveillance cells which are part of the acute inflammatory reaction). That vagal activity gives feedback to the macrophages, telling them to stop sending out inflammatory cytokine messengers.

Enter the Cholinergic Anti-inflammatory Pathway

This vagal feedback system was accurately but long-windedly named the cholinergic anti-inflammatory pathway by Dr. Kevin Tracey of New York's Feinstein Institutes for Medical Research and his colleagues in *Neuromodulation*. In the early 2000s, in animal studies, Tracey's group discovered that the vagus nerve activity through the α7nACh receptor could inhibit the potentially fatal inflammatory response to toxins resembling septic shock.[4]

Acetylcholine is the messenger or neurotransmitter produced by the vagus nerve. Tracey's group found that stimulating the vagus nerve could decrease inflammation more safely than intervening with acetylcholine or an acetylcholine equivalent, which would carry significant side effects.

Similarly, direct stimulation of the vagus nerve through implanted electrodes can also reduce inflammation in conditions like rheumatoid arthritis through the same pathways. Direct vagal nerve stimulation (which would *not* be considered a hormetic intervention in Dr. One's toolkit) harnesses the body's homeostatic feedback systems. While it has become big business, it has not been uniformly successful and there can be complications from the implantation process. Man is not a machine, even when tinkering with some of the most subtle levers.

But the finding that the α7nAChR receptor, this subunit

of the macrophage, is responsive to vagal stimulation gives us fascinating insight into the mechanisms behind Dr. One's methods. It tells us that this vagus-sensitive subunit is critical to acupuncture's effectiveness in suppressing inflammation. It also helps explain the benefits of other nonmedical interventions such as exercise, breathing, biofeedback and meditation. They can *all* stimulate vagal activity, which would increase rest-and-digest activity, and stimulate the α7nAChR receptors on macrophages, which decrease inflammatory cytokines.

Acupuncture and Anti-inflammatory Effects

Acupuncture on one of the most commonly used acupuncture points, Stomach 36, can reduce tumor necrosis factor (TNF), interleukin 6 (Il-6) and interleukin 1β (IL1-B) with mitigation of lung and kidney damage in septic rodents.[5]

Notably, the cytokine that *increased* in Dr. Tracey's original study was interleukin 10 (Il-10), an *anti*-inflammatory cytokine (not a pro-inflammatory cytokine like Il-6 and Il1-β.)[6] Interestingly, acupuncture stimulates an increase in IL-10, as does exercise, suggesting that both foster an environment of anti-inflammatory cytokines.

The hormetic of acupuncture *increases* anti-inflammatory messengers and *decreases* inflammatory messengers through the autonomic nervous system. It produces cascades of effects triggering the body's homeostatic mechanisms to achieve a global anti-inflammatory effect.

More Hormesis of Old Friends: Town versus Country

In Chapter 5, we discussed the phenomenon of "old friends." We saw how the removal of malarial parasites in Sardinia led to an overactive immune response in the island's inhabitants and an increase in autoimmune diseases. As unlikely as it sounds, the lack of other "old friends" such as animal dander and dirt can lead not only to an increase in the incidence of allergies, as the British witnessed in the 19th century, but also to increased stress, which, in turn, provokes inflammation.

Researcher Stefan Reber at the University of Ulm in Germany revealed the connection between good emotional health and growing up around dirt by comparing subjects who grew up in urban and rural environments. In his study, 40 men were put through a stress test in which they had to give a speech and solve complex math problems in front of stone-faced, white-coated scientists.[7] The men who grew up in cities without the benefit of being repeatedly challenged by a "dirty" hormetic environment showed exaggerated, prolonged elevation of the inflammatory compound interleukin 6 (Il-6), which persisted throughout the two-hour test period. Individuals raised in rural settings reported feeling stressed but did not show this dramatic increase in their inflammatory cytokines.

So, exposure to animals, dirt and dander is a hormetic challenge to the immune system that can prevent an overactive inflammatory response in the face of an intense psychological challenge. This might be a hard fact to wrap your head around. However, once we consider how the feedback systems in the body work, it becomes plausible. The immune challenge of dirt and animal dander reduces spikes in inflammation later in life. If you have a lower inflammatory reaction to a stress challenge, you are sturdier and less likely to spiral out of control.

Reber's human test subjects reacted similarly to the horses and beagles from the study in Chapter 3 did after their acupuncture treatment, registering the stress mentally but with little response in their inflammatory cytokines. If you recall, the beagles and horses in the study responded to startle in their reflex movements, but the acupuncture dampened their autonomic arousal. Human patients exposed to the hormetic challenges of dander growing up still experienced stress, but notably their inflammatory markers did not spike dramatically. Because of the nature of feedback systems, avoiding this provoked increase in inflammatory markers could be quite protective if extrapolated over years.

Radical Resilience and Prevention in Action

Given how our feedback systems amplify effects, you could argue that even avoiding one episode of increased inflammation could avert a vicious downward spiral. Avoiding an outsized reaction of our bodies with inflammation in the face of some inciting event is what we mean by radical resilience. If receiving acupuncture on an ongoing basis stabilizes your autonomic system enough to stay balanced when facing stressors, you wind up ahead. Even though the effect may be small, avoiding brief spikes in inflammation could ultimately be significant, since as we know, *it all spins together in a synergy of systems.* The point here is that we should not lock ourselves away so we never encounter any challenges. The overall goal is to make our system resilient enough to be able to face challenges and maintain balance. There are many ways to do this, including acupuncture, sauna, cold exposure and exercise.

Now that we can quantify these inflammatory flares with cytokines and our autonomic balance, we can see how this stability could provide potent prevention. We can understand how Dr. One's fame at "keeping his patients well" by treating *between* illnesses and injuries and nudging the body to stay ready to respond could be a true preventative. In animal research, this potential has been verified by studies that show animals given acupuncture and then injected with a substance causing sepsis had much better survival rates than those who did not get acupuncture. The effect appears to last for days—radical prevention in action. Now, our mental models have broadened to understand how this approach has validity. *Ancient wisdom, modern eyes.*

Getting Movement Through Balance

With this information in mind, let's revisit the case study of my patient BD. With her kind of stealth inflammation, acupuncture was able to help by stimulating her system and interrupting the vicious cycle of inflammation. Given what we know about acupuncture suppressing inflammatory cytokines, we should not be surprised at BD's successful treatment. Some evidence supporting this comes from animal studies that show electroacupuncture increases gut function and decreases inflammation through the α7nAChR pathway, the same one discovered by Dr. Tracey.[8] Since BD's inflammation was systemic, stimulating the vagus nerve with acupuncture helped improve her gut transit times and probably lessened her overall inflammation.[9]

This case illustrates the concept of radical resilience and how sturdy it is, just as in the study comparing farmers and city dwellers. Factors that used to throw off BD's regularity, such as travel and deadlines, do not do so anymore. Acupuncture has provided her stability in the face of challenges, the sort of radical prevention we seek. Through acupuncture, she dealt with her condition in a way that did not cause its own problems. Now, her gut brushes off stress and does its "business."

Keeping BD in mind, let's look at one of the most commonly used acupuncture points worldwide throughout the ages, a point that Dr. One would elect to use on her, as did I: Stomach 36.

Unlocking the Secrets of Acupuncture Points: The Remarkable Case of Stomach 36

Dr. One would use Stomach 36 for gastrointestinal conditions like constipation and to boost immunity in the case of an upper respiratory or other contagious illness. Stomach 36 is not near the stomach as you might imagine. It is actually located on the tibialis anterior, three inches below the kneecap. The ancient teaching is that patients will derive the most nourishment from their food by stimulating this point to strengthen the stomach, leading to robust health. Stomach 36 is also one of the most often used points in research on animals and humans. It is easy to find the analog point even in small animals.

Animal studies show that using acupuncture techniques on Stomach 36 increases stomach emptying and gut transit times (as in the case of BD), thereby alleviating constipation. One of these studies using acupuncture on Stomach 36 revealed decreased inflammatory markers via the vagus nerve and promoted gastrointestinal transit times through the α7nAChR pathway.[10] Another showed a similar triggering of the α7nAChR pathway in mice with induced acute pancreatitis.[11] This effect was clearly vagal in origin because the effect was erased when the vagus nerve was surgically removed. Both of these examples offer scientific evidence that the ancient practice of acupuncture provides a way to trigger the body's homeostatic healing mechanisms through vagal stimulation that Dr. Tracey and his colleagues initially sought.

New Research with Potential for More Reliable Results from Acupuncture

In all honesty, while acupuncture has tremendous potential, it doesn't always work, often requires multiple treatments and is not as reliable as practitioners might hope. However, a recent study provides clues as to how we may be able to improve acupuncture's results.

In a fascinating and groundbreaking development, research published in the prestigious journal *Nature*[12] found that Stomach 36 is close to a hindlimb nerve with specific markers (protein Prokr2). When these markers are found on a nerve, they predict whether that nerve will directly stimulate vagal activity. We know we provoke a general vagal effect needling the body, but this is more specific and powerful.

In their study, the researchers used optogenic stimulation on the acupuncture points instead of needles, a method that uses light to stimulate nerves. Through this method, the team not only identified other hindlimb nerves that had similarly increased potential for vagal stimulation, but also distinguished *which frequencies* of stimulation provided specific effects. Exploiting this remarkable finding is a way off from being able to be used in the clinic so precisely, but the potential could be enormous.

The study indicates that for centuries, Dr. One was using the correct point, Stomach 36, when tackling problems of gastrointestinal distress and improving immunity. The ancients had no idea they were triggering sophisticated immune response systems from the limbs to the brain and back to the vagus and macrophages, but this is precisely what they were doing. Modern science has taken the invisible and has made it visible.

Showing the Relationship between Autonomic Balance and Inflammation

Since increasing vagal activity can decrease inflammation, it would seem logical that a measure of overall vagal activity might correlate with an overall level of inflammation. As noted, we can evaluate the autonomic nervous system with heart rate variability (HRV). As a measure of stress, HRV turns out to be relevant to the inflammatory state of a person.[13] To illustrate with an example, rheumatoid arthritis, a chronic inflammatory state, has autonomic dysfunction and deterioration of HRV as a hallmark.

Rheumatoid Arthritis: A Body Out of Balance

The autonomic balance in rheumatoid arthritis (RA) patients is often unhealthy, with too much sympathetic fight-or-flight activity and insufficient vagal, rest-and-digest activity. But researchers are considering whether the autonomic imbalance is an inherent part of the disease and not a consequence of ongoing pain and disability as previously thought.

In one study, individuals at risk of RA who subsequently developed the condition had significantly higher resting heart rates than healthy subjects.[14] This finding accords with other studies, which reflect reduced parasympathetic nervous system activity or vagal activity, correlating with an impaired inflammatory reflex in patients with RA. The decline of the parasympathetic nervous system in RA precedes the manifestation of other disease classification criteria, such as joint involvement. This finding is consistent with the association between increased inflammatory status and decreased parasympathetic activity observed in healthy subjects in large studies.[15]

Another study looked at RA, autonomic balance and inflammatory markers and found that the lower and unhealthier the heart rate variability (HRV) of the subjects, the higher the inflammatory markers (Il-6 and C-reactive protein or CRP). These findings suggest that lower HRV is associated with increased inflammation and independently associated with increased pain in RA sufferers.[16] (Keep in mind that Il-6 is one of the inflammatory cytokines that *decreases* with acupuncture, as well as by direct vagal stimulation.)

In this context, Dr. Tracey's group's use of direct vagal stimulation is particularly appropriate. But of course, this is still a "cool toy." We could easily argue that noninvasive methods such as acupuncture, meditation and other interventions that increase parasympathetic activity may also help.

Even in young, healthy adults without RA, the levels of inflammatory markers (C-reactive protein and IL-6) are inversely related to HRV.[17] In addition, circulating tumor necrosis factor (TNF), another inflammatory cytokine, is an independent predictor of depressed HRV, reinforcing the concept of a close relationship between inflammation and the autonomic nervous system.[18]

Systems Synergy or "It All Spins Together"

In summary, we see that inflammation is a factor in many big killers including heart disease, cancer, dementia and even aging itself. But we also see the connection between too much sympathetic fight-or-flight activity and insufficient parasympathetic rest-and-digest activity leading to increased inflammation. Our mental framework is perhaps widening, enabling us to see how optimizing our own autonomic balance and other innate feedback systems can help fight a broad swath of ailments. Dr. One knew this, and now we can see the validity of this strategy through the most recent science.

Chapter 7
When Pain Strikes

"The easiest pain to bear is someone else's."
—Francois de la Rochefoucauld

"Of pain you could wish only one thing: that it should stop. Nothing in the world was so bad as physical pain. In the face of pain there are no heroes."
—George Orwell, *1984*

Susan's Story

Susan was a diligent, hyperactive senior executive at a prominent law firm. She was always on the go, but debilitating nerve pain in her feet had taken over her life. She'd been prescribed large doses of Neurontin (gabapentin) only to fall victim to a known side effect: a severe mood disorder making her depressed. Susan desperately needed to find a way to wean off Neurontin, as when she came to see me in the clinic, she was on the verge of suicide.

I treated Susan with both manual acupuncture and electroacupuncture twice a week. Within a month, her pain subsided. Her mood improved with acupuncture and after quitting the Neurontin. Though her pain flares if she's been on her feet for extended periods, it is now dramatically reduced, and she is fully functional again. She still comes weekly to the clinic because she wants to take no chances with her mood or the threat of disability from pain. She's joined a gym that helps with her overall biodynamics and enjoys activities with her young grandsons. Even though she's in her 70s, she continues to work full-time.

They say people fear pain more than death. But pain, even though it is universally feared, is still subject to the laws of Dr. One. Pain is affected directly by stress, mood and inflammation, so it can elude the sometimes dangerous "fix it" solutions provided by modern medicine. It is a clear example of how our bodies are not machines. Pain touches everyone from the cradle to the grave and takes a tremendous toll on the world. Some pain is unavoidable, and we do need good Dr. Twos to deal with it—but pain also gives us some of the clearest examples of the need for more Dr. Ones.

The importance of the law of balance and that we do no harm become clear when considering the hazards of back surgeries and opioids. The tyranny of bio-plausibility becomes obvious with cortisone injections, for example, which are very popular but need to be used with care. Because pain and its perception rely on feedback loops, it is one of many biological systems that best illustrates the nature of *nonlinearity* where cause and effect are not always proportional. Small or even nonexistent stimuli can lead to an exaggerated perception of pain, while conversely, severe pain sometimes isn't perceived at all.

Similarly, the model of *man-as-machine* doesn't serve us when abnormal X-rays and MRIs are inconsistent with the degree of patients' back pain. Following the law of systems synergy, there's a biochemical connection between stress and pain, and elements of the immune system are intimately related to pain and its perception.

In this chapter, we'll explore the daunting challenge of pain. We will consider the horrible burden of pain on patients and society, and how the warning of "do no harm" comes into stark relief when looking at the horror of the opiate crisis. We'll see how nonlinearity—that nonproportionality of cause and effect—comes into full display when pain becomes chronic. Treating chronic pain requires careful treatment that takes into account how stress and our immune health are closely correlated to our experience of pain. Along the way, we'll learn how two patients, in addition to Susan, overcame their pain conditions with acupuncture. But first, let's start with the scope of society's pain problem and some of the hazards of current medical solutions.

Scope of the Problem of Pain

Pain is terrifying for patients, challenging for the medical profession and one of the most common conditions seen in acupuncture clinics. It is a major health problem with horrific social and economic consequences that costs the US economy between $560 billion and $635 billion annually in physician visits, analgesics and lost productivity. That's the equivalent of $1,706 to $1,934 for every man, woman and child.[1]

Do No Harm: The Toll of the Opioid Crisis

Besides the costs and disabilities of pain, the related opioid crisis has caused a massive increase in misery and expense. Every day, more than 1,000 people are treated in emergency departments for misusing *prescription* opiates obtained from various Dr. Twos. Consider the following statistics from the Center for Disease Control:

- In 2021, there were an estimated 107,622 drug overdose deaths in the US, an increase of 15 percent over the previous year. (To put that in perspective: 58,000 US military personnel were killed in 19 years of the Vietnam War.)

- Overdose deaths involving opioids increased from 70,029 in 2020 to 80,816 in 2021.
- Overdoses involving prescription opioids were responsible for 16,419 deaths in 2020.
- In 2019, an estimated 10.1 million people aged 12 or older misused opioids.
- The CDC estimates that the US's total economic burden of prescription opioid misuse is $78.5 billion a year, including health care costs, lost productivity, addiction treatment and criminal justice involvement.
- Eighty percent of people who use heroin first misused prescription opiates. [2]

Big Pharma is involved in any medical condition that has a massive market, which means pain is big business. In Chapter 2, we saw how this played out with disastrous effects for baseball player Micah Bowie. When it comes to pain management, the risk-to-benefit ratio can be enormous. Can the ancients *really* teach us anything about mitigating pain and keeping the patient from spiraling out of control?

As discussed, doctors face overwhelming pressures to treat medical conditions (to "do something"), and pain is no exception. The opioid crisis is a stunning example. Derived from poppies, opiates apparently evolved with us since we have specific receptors for them. Those same receptors habituate very quickly, however, requiring ever greater dosages to maintain the same level of pain relief. Deaths from overdoses have reached every community, from major urban centers to remote rural towns. Many of these tragedies start and end with medications requiring a doctor's prescription.

How did we reach the point where so many doctors have

fallen into the Dr. Three category? It goes back to the late 1990s when healthcare providers began prescribing opioid pain relievers at greater rates. The pharmaceutical companies reassured physicians that patients would not become addicted. Even today, doctors often prescribe opioids for relatively benign conditions such as a sprained ankle or post-operative pain. But once patients start taking them, the *physical* need for more opioids arises to remain in equilibrium and avoid withdrawal. It can happen to anyone, not only those that are genetically predisposed. While not all opioid addiction is from medical prescriptions, a massive amount of needless suffering and death has been visited on the public by an army of Dr. Twos who degenerated into Dr. Threes. But it didn't start with them. Often, the Dr. Threes were pushed by the "pushers" at Big Pharma who were following the money.

Perhaps the most egregious example is Purdue Pharma, the makers of OxyContin, a popular and wildly overprescribed opioid. After a lengthy legal battle, the company's owners, the Sackler family, agreed to pay up to $6 billion to settle thousands of opioid-related lawsuits.[3] Though that sounds good, the amount was utterly inadequate. The Sackler's insisted all civil-related claims be dropped. They insisted that they be granted immunity from liability. They insisted that they be allowed 18 years to pay their $1 billion compensation to victims. Under the bankruptcy plan, the Sackler's' money, plus billions more from the company, would be distributed to states, municipalities and tribes to treat and prevent opioid addiction and compensate victims. Justice delayed is justice denied.

Neurontin, the Stealth Destabilizer

Another example of a widely prescribed drug for pain is Neurontin, the medication that drove my patient Susan to contemplate suicide. Initially developed for seizure disorders,

Neurontin has had an eyebrow-raising run as an "off-label" medication for everything from restless leg syndrome to migraines. Perhaps the cleverest thing that the developers did was to name this anti-seizure medication Neurontin. That way, there was bio-plausibility in prescribing it for nerve issues.

As I've seen in the clinic, there can be distressing side effects even when Neurontin is taken as prescribed. In many instances, it doesn't help at all. Neurontin can be what I call a "stealth destabilizer." Because it's not a controlled substance, any Dr. Two can prescribe Neurontin in large doses, and it is relatively inexpensive if you have insurance. It has also likely contributed to the opioid crisis because it can enhance the effects of opioids. Employees taking both opiates and Neurontin may pass required workplace drug testing and still be impaired on the job. Workers high on drugs in the workplace can lead to safety hazards for themselves and others. There are even withdrawal symptoms from the supposedly non-addictive Neurontin, the most common being agitation and confusion. When stealth destabilizers lead to the ultimate spiraling out of control, causing patients to consider suicide, you know you need to use caution.

Cortisone Shots: A Quick Pain Reliever at What Cost?

The body produces corticosteroids under stress in response to inflammation. Steroid injections can quickly relieve joint inflammation with effects lasting from several weeks to several months. This has made them popular as a "quick fix," but while I've seen several patients who enjoyed significant relief through steroid injections, many others have no relief. Some recent research came to some concerning conclusion about cortisone joint injections for osteoarthritis of the hip or knee: there's no compelling evidence that they work.[4] In fact, the injections *worsened* conditions for seven to eight percent of patients, whose arthritis accelerated "beyond the expected rate." Unusual fractures or bone damage (osteonecrosis) may occur in about one percent of people in both conditions as well; other side effects include a temporary increase in blood sugar, bleeding into the joint and in rare instances, infection.

In Chapter 2, we saw in the Bowie example the extreme spiraling out of control that invasive pain treatment can cause. Similarly, the overprescription of opioids has caused tremendous suffering and death, and Neurontin caused a distressing case of a severe mood disorder in my patient Susan,. Even corticosteroids, so commonly used and considered safe, can cause worsening arthritis and other problems. As all these examples show, Dr. Twos can easily slide into becoming Dr. Threes.

Do No Harm: Hazards of Back Procedures and Surgeries

Back Surgeries

Though there are some high-profile cases of successful back surgery, alas, more often than not, it doesn't work. In 2019, Tiger Woods had a successful spinal fusion that prompted Dartmouth spine surgeon Dr. Sohail K. Mirza to say that such a positive outcome was so rare it was "like winning the lottery." And two years later, Tiger needed back surgery again —his fifth.[5] Granted, the torque and stress placed on a golfer's back are extreme and Woods needed help, but back surgery is common even though it has a poor track record.

In the *man-as-machine* model, back surgery *should* work. Unfortunately, it often doesn't and can make matters worse. Of course, *interventionista* doctors are paid $80,000 to $150,000 for this surgery, which is a significant amount (*follow the money*)! That amount would easily pay for a year of acupuncture and physical therapy, a limo ride to and from the clinic, a nice lunch afterward and cleaning services for your home. Of course, in the US, health insurance would never pay for any of that, unlike Germany, where medical insurers at least cover spa treatments.[6]

Dr. Charles A. Reitman, co-director of the Spine Center at the Medical University of South Carolina, says there can be decent results from fusion back surgery for people who suffer a broken spine, scoliosis (severe spinal curvature) or spondylolisthesis, in which vertebrae slip out of place: "If you look at it simplistically, what does fusion do? It provides mechanical support. If they are missing mechanical support and that is the pure cause of the problem, then they will get better."[7] But most fusion procedures are because of degenerated disks that are worn out, dehydrated, stiff and friable.

Disabling lower back pain from degenerated disks often improves on its own even though the disk is still degenerated, although it's unclear why. To add to the confusion, about half of middle-aged people with no back pain have degenerated disks, and at least half of patients in pain who have a fusion for a degenerated disk remain in pain. Dartmouth's Dr. Mirza says the surgeries aren't worth it: "If your goal is cure, that isn't what this is going to offer."

Regardless, fusion surgery is among the top five operations in the US, and the vast majority are performed for deteriorated disks. Only knee and hip replacements account for more inpatient hospital stays. Medicare pays for 300,000 of these operations each year, and private insurers pay for about the same amount. That number represents the equivalent of performing back surgery on every citizen of Vermont.

Another option for patients willing to be, well, patient, is intensive physical therapy. Large clinical trials have found that as a group, those who take this route have outcomes indistinguishable from those who have surgery. Still, it must be the right kind of physical therapy to strengthen back muscles and improve flexibility (using the principle of hormesis).

So, what can Dr. One offer? How can acupuncture and other solutions help treat pain conditions?

Chinese Medicine's Pain Theories Made Modern

In the ancient classic *The Yellow Emperor*, author Huangdi Neijing writes:

> *Where there is movement, there is no pain. When the qi [pronounced "chee," roughly defined as energy] and blood flowing continuously through the body within the channels are attacked by a cold pathogen, they stagnate. If the cold pathogen attacks outside the channels in the periphery, it will simply decrease the blood flow. When it attacks within the channels, it blocks the qi flow and creates pain.*[8]

As the passage above explains, in Chinese medicine, musculoskeletal pain represents a "stagnation pattern" in the meridians and causes pain. Physical therapy in Western medicine incorporates similar principles. Physical therapy aims to increase flexibility and strength in corresponding and complementary muscles to increase function and relieve pain, hence the orthopedic adage, "motion is lotion." If you can decrease the pain, you can get more mobility, motion, blood flow and function. This means you get less "stagnation" leading to less pain. Acupuncture, massage and heat can also help reduce stagnation and engender a virtuous, feed-forward cycle of healing.

To fully understand the underlying science of these alternative pain treatments, let's briefly consider the two general types of pain: acute pain, which is more linear and easier to understand and treat, and chronic conditions that are nonlinear and can be challenging to treat.

Acute Pain: Here Today and Gone Tomorrow

In ancient times, Dr. Ones and Dr. Twos might treat acute pain for a pulled muscle or strained ligament with direct needling, massage or calming teas. Of course, any serious accident would require more drastic interventions like primitive types of surgery and medications or the application of splints with the hope that the person will heal once repaired and stabilized.

To this day, urgent acute situations need aggressive surgery and powerful medications, because their benefits far outweigh the significant risks. Dr. Twos play a massive role in these serious circumstances. We are blessed to have the miracles of modern medicine like trauma centers, blood transfusions and powerful medications. But what happens when healing does not occur? That is the challenge of chronic pain that can happen with or without preceding surgery.

Chronic Pain: The Ongoing Thorn in Your Side

To understand the more complicated—and in some instances, intractable—problem of chronic pain, I'll provide a brief overview of how pain is transmitted. Pain usually starts in the periphery (the peripheral nervous system) with nociceptors or pain receptors. They relay the pain message to the spinal column and then up to the brain, which comprise the central nervous system. The brain processes the information as pain and then feeds back to the periphery to heal the injury. Multiple pathways are involved in this "top-down" feedback, from anti-inflammatory processes to hormonal systems. One of the pathways is my "favorite" feedback system, the conduit of the autonomic nervous system.

We are all vulnerable to imbalance and dysfunction in pain perception due to the unique interactions of genetic (anterior heaven), epigenetic (posterior heaven) and environmental factors. Because of this, some chronic pain conditions can be the product of system imbalance. Research from Dr. James Rainville, a physical medicine specialist in Boston's New England Baptist Hospital, back pain "often has nothing to do with the mechanics of the spine, but with the way the nervous system is behaving." As he explains:

> *About 25 percent of patients with acute back trouble get stuck in an endless loop of pain often due to persistent hypersensitivity of the nervous system, a change in how the sensory system processes information. Normal sensations of touch, sensations produced by movements, are translated by the nervous system into a pain message. That process is what drives people completely crazy who have back pain because so many things produce discomfort.* [9]

As Dr. Rainville's explanation shows us once again, man is not a machine—and input does not equal output.

False Signals

We think of pain in terms of linear cause and effect: You hurt yourself, and the pain is your body's way of telling you something is wrong and to stop what you're doing right now. But for some people, that pain is a false signal. "It's not about looming danger; it's actually caused by hypersensitive nerves," says Dr. Rainville. [10]

Athletes, Soldiers and the Paradox of Pain

The pathway from the periphery to the brain and back is what makes pain so subjective, as various inputs can interfere with the loop. In athletes or soldiers, for example, powerful fight-or-flight reflexes can override the brain's pain impulses. It's why that same complicated feedback loop system allows athletes to keep playing despite a severe injury during a crucial game.

This lack of symmetry can work in reverse too: a person can have a normal back X-ray but be feeling excruciating pain. This lack of correlation between X-rays and pain is also why back surgeries have a dismal track record—despite their perceived value which comes from being expensive, cool and very bio-plausible.

When Pain Is "All in the Head"

Sometimes long after an original injury has healed, intractable, chronic and unrelenting pain remains because the brain has been thrown out of balance and continues to relay pain signals. Sometimes the brain even engages more brain "real estate" to react to this non-impulse through a process called central sensitization, making it feel more severe. In some ways, the pain really is "all in the head," but that does not mean it is fake or that the patient is malingering or making things up.

Central sensitization is a system out of balance, an asymmetry of perception. In patients where this has happened, perhaps the initial wildfire of pain has subsided. The tissues may even be healed. But the pain can remain or even ramp up. In these cases, the mental models of *man-as-machine* and proportionality of input equal an output breakdown. Since the injury is no longer there, it should be "fixed"—yet the pain remains and resists numbing with local anesthetics at the wound site or even spinal anesthesia. The pain comes from the brain in a feedback loop that has spiraled out of control. It is challenging for modern practitioners to treat.

As in Susan's case, chronic pain can also be caused by peripheral neuropathy. Dr. One's acupuncture can provide an effective alternative, however, with a needling strategy for which there is now scientific evidence.

Beyond the Gate: The Evolving Science of Acupuncture's Secrets

When I started my acupuncture practice, the prevailing scientific model for acupuncture's effectiveness was called "gating," a theory popularized by researchers Ronald Melzack and Patrick Wall. Gating suggests you can occupy pain receptors or "gates" with non-painful stimuli like rubbing, vibration or small needles,[11] reducing pain.[12] A simple example of gating is when you accidentally hit your head on something and instinctively rub the spot. Rubbing occupies the pain receptors competing in the spinal canal for the pain signals to the brain.

It is worth noting that this natural reaction to acute pain *does* help, and gating remains an important model for acupuncture's pain-relieving effects. But as we now know, gating is far from the only mechanism of action. If it were, then acupressure, tapping or similar modalities that occupy the pain receptors would be enough.

Cross Talk, Feedback and the Role of the Immune System

Mast Cells Orchestrating Inflammation and Pain

In the decades since the pioneering work of Melzack and Wall, modern science has delivered an extensive body of research detailing the neurotransmitters, cytokines and other biochemical compounds that modify how pain is perceived, modified and alleviated. As we've seen and will continue to explore, the systems are all interrelated. A remarkable example of Dr. One's law comes from studying the neuroimmune interface, the interaction of nerves and pain with the immune system.

As discussed in Chapter 5, there are cells that reside in

various tissues that constitute the first line of host defense analogous to Metchnikoff's "wandering cells." They are known as *mast cells*, and they release multiple messengers affecting the immune system, vascular system and growth factors in response to allergens, viruses and bacteria. Because of their proximity to blood vessels and nerve fibers, mast cells are major players in orchestrating inflammation-associated pain.[13]

Mast cells are crucial to the potency of acupuncture points and may explain some of the more curious experiences associated with needling. Some of these responses include the appearance of a reddening around the inserted needle or the sensation of itching. There is also a curious phenomenon called *de qi*, a feeling of heaviness that some patients encounter. These intriguing effects give us some clues as to what, besides gating, might explain acupuncture's effectiveness.

Though electroacupuncture is widespread in practice and research, it does not activate mast cells to the same extent as manual acupuncture. The activation of mast cells is more intense with mechanical stimulation. This finding reinforces the time-honored usefulness of a few traditional techniques in ancient acupuncture, such as rotating and manipulating the needles. There can even be a sensation of a "grabbing" of the needle (traditionally called "catching a fish") resulting from the interaction of the needle with collagen fibers, which explains why "rougher" needles disturb more of the tissues involved and often work better.[14]

From Bites to Needles: An Evolutionary Response

We know from animal experiments that needling is analogous to a bite or splinter from an evolutionary standpoint. The body reacts with macrophages and cytokines, stimulating an immune response in the periphery. The minor injury of needling ultimately leads to a *decrease* in inflammatory markers and less pain, mediated through the autonomic nervous system and other homeostatic systems. This primary feedback pathway through the autonomic nervous system includes sympathetic and parasympathetic fibers. The autonomic nervous system increases vagal, rest-and-digest activity and decreases fight-or-flight, which reduces inflammation, induces relaxation and improves blood flow.

The body gets hormetically challenged at regular intervals during ongoing acupuncture treatment. These repeated challenges calm the body, improving vagal activity and promoting better mood and sleep. Better sleep leads to improved healing and less pain, and the virtuous cycle of healing is set into motion. The small input of needling gets outsized or asymmetric results—an example of the system's nonlinearity due to feed-forward loops. Ancient doctors were correct, in a way. By seeing pain as "stagnation" and using needles to "unblock the meridians," they unwittingly stimulated a cascade of self-correcting and healing homeostatic mechanisms by introducing a slight but real injury.

The Intricate Link between Stress and Pain

Research shows that increased stress can affect most types of pain, from migraine to back pain. As discussed, an increase in fight-or-flight activity can override pain signals when pain is acute. However, if fight-or-flight persists, it can worsen pain because of vagal withdrawal (a decrease in rest-and-digest activity), causing an increase in inflammation. For example, as shown by a study mentioned in Chapter 6, if you remove the vagus nerve (the autonomic nervous system's conduit for rest-and-digest activity) from mice treated with acupuncture for induced colitis, the mice exhibit more pain than the control group whose vagus nerves are intact. This study shows that at least *some* of acupuncture's pain-killing effect is through the autonomic nervous system, the vagus nerve in particular.[15]

As Dr. Joseph Audette, a clinical acupuncturist, puts it, "Acupuncture also has a dramatic effect on your nervous system, calming you down so your body can rejuvenate faster. It's basically what's supposed to happen when you meditate, except it's even stronger and faster. Acupuncture relaxes your muscles, slows your heart rate and reduces inflammation to promote healing."[16]

This stress-lowering effect works for immune function, inflammation and pain syndromes, too. In the clinic, when a patient's overall stress level decreases, it leaves them resistant to recurrences and other stressors, the sort of radical resilience and prevention that is the hallmark of Dr. One. But let's consider further implications of how this works.

Decreased inflammation means that a patient might require less medication, leading to fewer side effects and a more balanced system that is less likely to spiral out of control. By understanding this, we see that Dr. One's advice to manage stress, sleep well and lead a balanced life *can* help with pain management and lead to fewer vicious, feed-forward cycles of pain. Dr. One would, of course, give acupuncture, but other means are at everyone's disposal: meditation, breathing techniques, massage and being in nature can all increase parasympathetic activity and help create a state of calm with many health benefits.[17]

In Susan's case, being able to wean off Neurontin improved her mood. It enabled her to live normally, feel optimistic enough to continue her treatments and ultimately prevail over her condition. But let me introduce you to KU, another patient of mine, who had been having debilitating back pain for a year before coming to see me.

KU's Story: Needles over Knives

KU was a slender, bookish academic who'd had debilitating back pain for a year, and sitting for any length of time was difficult for him. The exercise he loved the most, swimming, only aggravated the pain. So did physical therapy. His orthopedic surgeon suggested surgery, but for a person like KU, the risk-to-benefit of surgery wasn't particularly favorable. KU was still functional if not optimally functional; surgery could make things better, but if it didn't, it could also make them a lot worse. Ultimately, he declined surgery and came to me seeking an alternative solution of acupuncture, which made more sense and had less risk.

When I began to treat KU with acupuncture, I discovered he was extremely sensitive to needling, so I used the finest, thinnest needles. After a few visits, although the pain wasn't completely gone, he could walk farther distances and felt cautiously encouraged. He made so much progress that he could even fulfill a planned trip to Greece, which excited him as a Classics scholar and professor. He was able to withstand the plane trip, the general rigor of travel and carrying his baggage. Europe can be challenging because of the cobblestones, uneven surfaces and the frequent need to walk great distances. But in spite of a rigorous itinerary, he still managed and was overjoyed. A series of acupuncture sessions was able to ease KU's pain, improve his mobility and dramatically decrease his disability.

By keeping KU's story in mind, our mental models start to shift to include the concept of nonlinearity, as a subtle intervention with needles lead him to life-changing results. By employing the laws of doing no harm and the gentle hormesis of needling, we were able to achieve a virtuous cycle of healing. But is there room in our thinking for this quite radical idea?

Back pain can be a vicious cycle of poor function and

muscle tension leading to decreased blood flow. As Dr. One would say, "stagnation" can lead to a chronic pain condition where even minimal movement hurts. The body has ceased to address the pain. In a sense, it is walled off. Needles stimulate the body to heal. On entry, they cause the aggregation of local immune cells. The pain receptors send signals through the periphery to the central nervous system, which then sends signals back down to the area to decrease inflammatory substances and increase endorphins. In addition to overall vagal improvement, needles in the area help direct this action so the immune messengers will go where the needles are placed.

The reaction around the needles helps ease the "stagnation" until the pain decreases enough for the patient to move more freely. The freer movement around the site of pain leads to more blood flow and subsequent better function, leading to even *more* movement. This is a virtuous feed-forward cycle taking advantage of the principle that "motion is lotion." All of this shows that needling can reverse the vicious cycle of restricted movement, poor blood flow and more pain leading to less movement, hypersensitization of the brain and then even *less* movement. All of is made possible by using Dr. One's principles of balance and doing no harm.

Expanding Mental Models: Accepting Nonlinearity

Nonlinearity

Demanding a solution for pain commensurate with the degree of pain can lead to problems, as we've seen. Because of our intense fear of pain and the level of disability it can cause, there's a natural tendency to want the "big guns" as a solution. There is also the urgent pressure to "do something" (the *interventionista* mindset). Using the "big guns" can mean "strong medicine" (prescription drugs), the newest surgeries (cool toys), expensive specialists (the "smartest doctors") and bio-plausible solutions. Unfortunately, the more desperation there is, the more likely the patient and their doctor will spiral out of control, making a Dr. Two deteriorate into Dr. Three.

But remember: more is not always more. And from the perspective of complexity science and the law of nonlinearity, inputs do *not* always equal outputs. This is the pitfall of the inadequate mental model of proportionality, where input must be proportional to output. People see pain as a simple equation: you sprain an ankle, you heal and then it's over. Right? Often, that assumption can be right. Over-the-counter medications or physical therapy can be good enough for acute pain. But chronic pain can be much more complicated.

The main takeaway is that pain is not a simple system, even in the case of direct cause (injury) and effect (pain perception). It can be a distressing negative cycle where mood affects stress, stress affects pain and pain affects mood. But this vicious cycle also gives us an opening to disrupt it and turn it into a positive one. Keeping that in mind, let's use another patient story to consider a disabling but non-life-threatening type of pain that afflicts millions of Americans: migraine.

OC's Story: Relief from Migraines

One of my patients who I'll call OC is the head of one of the largest institutions in San Francisco. Not only has he overseen new construction of the organization's flagship space, but as director, he also needs to be responsive to major donors and trustees while overseeing special events and acquisitions. He takes his responsibility to employees very seriously and functions at an extremely high level. He constantly traveled worldwide despite suffering as many as three migraine attacks a week—often triggered by poor sleep, another chronic condition he endured.

Migraine is one of the most intense non-life-threatening pain syndromes, characterized by searing pain in the head (often behind the eyes) and requiring sufferers to retreat to a darkened room to sleep. Sometimes migraines are accompanied by vomiting or preceded by an "aura" that warns of the oncoming torment.

OC managed his stress by being an avid cyclist and devotee of spin classes, but it wasn't enough. Usually, he just "worked through" the migraines but with misery and loss of productivity. Other migraine patients are completely incapacitated, and their work, weekends and family life suffer incalculably. But how does a condition like migraine, which is so disabling, respond to some gentle needling?

OC came to see me at his wife's urging and diligently kept his appointments. Interestingly, migraine patients are often organized and meticulous—personality traits characteristic of a liver condition in Chinese medicine often thought to lead to migraines. In those teachings, some migraines are considered an imbalance of excess yang in the head and liver stagnation, among other etiologies. Since migraine patients typically have a hypersensitive system to all kinds of inputs from food to smells to light, treating them with acupuncture can be tricky. Sometimes, the treatment itself can trigger a migraine.[18] But to use acupuncture as hormesis, we need to nudge the body enough to get it accustomed to triggers. As we have seen, the needling invokes a cascade of healing responses, including increased vagal activity.

I encouraged OC to restrict his use of medications since they can keep the system out of balance. I measured his sympathetic and parasympathetic activity with heart rate variability (HRV) monitoring and saw a consistent decrease within each treatment and over weeks to months. After six treatments, we started to see real results. His migraines dropped from three a week to once a month or less. He kept up with monthly visits and then tapered to quarterly visits, and his migraines remain under control. Travel had always been extremely difficult for OC because of time zone changes, poor sleep and intense responsibility. But, for the most part, the intermittent hormetic challenge of the needles and the calming of the nervous system has helped him become sturdier and stronger. He now takes the rigors of traveling in stride.

Medications, of course, are often required for severe migraines. But if these treatments are minimized, the overall rate of migraines can be lower, as the system is less reactive. Many migraine medications can cause "rebound headaches" when the drug wears off, which can require more medication, keeping the patient's system out of balance. It's why, when patients first come in for an acupuncture visit saying that they don't take medications because they don't work for them or they simply don't want to, I feel like my job is more than halfway done.

Systems Synergy and How "It All Spins Together"

In summary, even in the bleak world of pain, there are ways to engage our feedback systems and interrupt things from spiraling out of control. Some of our chemical messengers can be nudged from the skin to the brain and back to decrease inflammation and the misfiring of nerves and pain. Doing no harm can also be crucial to averting disaster in pain syndromes, which means considering the significant roles that the immune system and inflammation play in the feedback loops affecting pain. Finally, stress can also worsen all types of pain because of decreases in vagal activity. But interrupting these feedback systems with small interventions can sometimes lead to outsized radical resilience.

Chapter 8
Mood Disorders: Dissolving the Mind/Body Barrier

"The so-called 'psychotically depressed' person who tries to kill herself [does so] the same way a trapped person will eventually jump from the window of a burning high-rise. Make no mistake about people who leap from burning windows. . . . You'd have to have personally been trapped and felt flames to really understand a terror way beyond falling."

—David Foster Wallace, *Infinite Jest*

Laura's Story from *The New Yorker*

Laura was a brilliant young woman who ended up on multiple medications after a diagnosis of bipolar disease. She almost dropped out of Harvard and tried to commit suicide. Laura was on 14 medications in three years and gained 40 pounds. She likely would have become homeless if she had not come from an affluent family.

During outpatient treatment after her suicide attempt, Laura's pharmacologist prescribed naltrexone, a drug believed to block the craving for alcohol. This was in addition to the antidepressant Effexor, Lamictal (anti-epileptic), Seroquel (an antipsychotic), Abilify (an antipsychotic), Ativan (a benzodiazepine for anxiety), lithium (for bipolar disorder and suicide prevention) and Synthroid, a medication to treat hypothyroidism (a side effect of lithium). She was so sedated by the drug combo that she sometimes slept 14 hours a night.

In an extensive *New Yorker* article, writer Rachel Aviv chronicled the harrowing process that patients go through trying to quit antidepressant drugs, partly by relating Laura's experience. Aviv reported how Rachel's pharmacologist had her stop taking Ativan first and Abilify a few weeks later. Aviv wrote that, "[Laura] began sweating so much that she could wear only black. If she turned her head quickly, she felt woozy. Her body ached, and occasionally she was overwhelmed by waves of nausea. Cystic acne broke out on her face and her neck. Her skin pulsed with a strange kind of energy." Later, she quotes Laura as saying, "I never felt quiet in my body. It felt like there was a current of some kind under my skin, and I was trapped inside this encasing that was constantly buzzing."

A month later, Laura discontinued Effexor, but her fear of people judging her circled inside her head. Like so many others, Laura thought that depression was the result of a chemical imbalance in the brain which her medications would recalibrate—until she researched and discovered that Big Pharma's theory was not backed by evidence. She also found that few studies outlined how to ease off the antidepressant meds. She was feeling horrible and struggling to figure it out on her own.

In this chapter, we will explore how the new science behind mood disorders provides some hope for new therapies. You'll learn that the fabric behind the theory of an imbalance in brain chemistry as the source of depression is gossamer thin. We will see how mood is tightly related to autonomic balance and it has an inflammatory component. We will consider whether vagal stimulation may be part of the answer. We will discover how the ancient Dr. One was correct in assessing the mind and body as inseparable and how his techniques to maintain balance benefit mood, just as they've benefited immune balance, pain, stress and longevity.

Scope of the Problem

Depression is cause for deep concern because the incidence of depression is extraordinarily high. Depression and suicide go hand in hand, and according to a 2019 report from the World Health Organization (WHO), one in every 100 deaths worldwide that year was a result of suicide.[1] Depression disrupts the workplace, family life and school commitments. Tragically, the lives of seven percent of men and one percent of women with a lifetime history of depression end in suicide. Clearly, depression is a disorder that warrants serious attention.

Medical expenditures for depression are on a scale similar to those for stroke, and in the US, its absenteeism costs are higher than those of type 2 diabetes.[2] Anxiety is the yang to depression's yin and contributes to the overall burden of what are loosely considered "mood disorders." While some consider these conditions "all in the head" or even a personal failing, they represent very real and costly medical conditions.

The "Science" behind Selective Serotonin Uptake Inhibitors or SSRIs

The pharmaceutical industry's solution was the development of the selective serotonin reuptake inhibitor (SSRI) class of antidepressants—the first and most famous being Prozac, which earned the nickname "bottled sunshine." The US Food and Drug Administration approved the drug to treat depression in 1987, and by 2019, there were more than 27 million prescriptions annually for over five million patients.[3]

Historically, the rationale underpinning the efficacy of SSRIs is the "monoamine-depletion hypothesis," in which an imbalance, mainly between serotonergic and noradrenergic neurotransmission, is proposed to be the basis of major depressive disorder. However, this "chemical imbalance" alone cannot fully explain the pathology and is far from proven.[4] Physicians confess to using it as a convenient shorthand way to explain it to patients.

As is often said in medicine, once a theory is out there, it's too late to rethink it. We saw Dr. Rita Redberg call this phenomenon "once the train has left the station" in Chapter 2. Unfortunately, Big Pharma has promoted the idea of chemical imbalances to such an extent that it has become ingrained in our thinking. Patients are relieved to hear they have a "real" illness that can be "fixed." In the *man-as-machine* model, Dr. Twos (the *interventionistas*) can swoop into action to "fix" the problem with prescription drugs like Prozac.

The chemical imbalance diagnosis operates somewhat similarly to how X-rays relate to back pain. As discussed earlier, X-rays are often red herrings to the actual problem causing someone's back pain. Once a problem is X-ray visible, it opens the door to the bio-plausibility of surgery or medication that can cure it. Equally, once the physician floats the comforting diagnosis of chemical imbalance as the cause of depression, patients grasp it in the hope of alleviating their suffering.

Multiple homeostatic feedback systems in the body are involved with mood, as they are with so many other conditions. The immune system and inflammatory response are involved in depression; so, too, is the autonomic nervous system and heart rate variability (HRV). These physical inputs directly affect conditions that are supposedly "all in the head." Just as the ancients described, the whole body is involved. Sadly, many patients don't consider breathing, acupuncture or yoga as first-line treatments for depression since they have been led to believe their brains need "fixing" with medication.

First, Do No Harm: The First Law of Balance

Given the overall burden to society in medical and other costs, you would think that depression would be under control, but that is far from the case. Depression can be tough to treat, and treatment itself can sometimes lead to a devolution of Dr. Twos into Dr. Threes, leading to an ultimate destabilization resulting in suicide.

Given the high rate of people who suffer from depression and its vicious cycle of multiple medications and side effects make an excellent case for considering Dr. One's remedies. Other mild and severe mood disorders are beyond this book's scope. Anxiety, for instance, has its own issues and anti-anxiety medications with their own side effects.

The Challenges of SSRI Antidepressants

SSRIs can be complicated to prescribe. There are quite a few to choose from and it can take weeks to see if they work. And by then, it's entirely possible the patient would have gotten better anyway. If a medication doesn't work, the process is to taper off its use, try a different one or add one and wait again for weeks to gauge the outcome. This is a lengthy and dicey process—dicey because antidepressants have the dubious distinction of possibly causing the very problem they're trying to cure. In some cases, with extreme consequences.

As discussed, suicide risk can increase when people take SSRIs (making antidepressants a treatment in the Dr. Three category). Other side effects include sexual dysfunction, insomnia, anxiety and anorexia. There is also a chance SSRIs will make you gain weight,[5] though the medical profession did not admit weight gain as a side effect for at least a decade.[6] In my clinic, I have seen many dumbfounded patients who gained 30 pounds within a few months of initiating antidepressant medications. Of course, these cases are not universal, but it catches your attention. After all, sudden and dramatic weight gain certainly doesn't help anybody's state of mind.

As far back as the 1990s, people have filed lawsuits blaming Prozac for violent behavior or suicidal tendencies. More recently, others have filed lawsuits for Prozac allegedly causing congenital disabilities in their children.[7]

The misery of depression can be compounded by medications that may not work, the possibility of debilitating side effects, weight gain and even suicide. Yet these drugs are still hugely popular. So, how did we get here? Unsurprisingly, some of the culprits for their widespread use, despite their meager success, are the same as those behind the prevalence of back surgery. We are now well familiar with "following the money", dodgy profit incentives, the *interventionista* mindset, sketchy research and flouting the warning to "do no harm," are all at play here.

Following the Money

The market for mood enhancers is enormous, and where there is money to be made, there are perverse incentives. Antidepressant research is a textbook example of burying negative results.[8] According to researchers who examined the results of 70 double-blind, placebo-controlled trials, suicidal thoughts and aggressive behavior doubled in children and adolescents who took two common types of antidepressants: SSRIs and serotonin and norepinephrine reuptake inhibitors (SNRIs).[9]

A study in the *Journal of Clinical Epidemiology* revealed that pharma employees, not independent researchers, wrote a third of the meta-analyses of the antidepressant studies.[10] And these pharma-backed studies were 22 times less likely than other meta-studies to include negative statements about the drug. What a surprise! Joanna Moncrieff, a psychiatrist and researcher at University College London, told *Scientific American*, "My view is that we really don't have good enough evidence that antidepressants are effective, and we have increasing evidence that they can be harmful, so we need to go into reverse and stop this increasing trend of prescribing [them]."[11]

Another vexing phenomenon is that major surgery and some prescription and non-prescription medications can lead to depression. In my practice, it has been devastating to witness patients have successful surgeries but then spiral into a major depression afterwards. In some cases, patients can be mentally affected for years after major surgery.

According to University of Illinois at Chicago researchers, about 200 prescription drugs can cause depression. The list includes common medications like proton pump inhibitors (PPIs) used to treat acid reflux, beta-blockers for high blood pressure, birth control pills and emergency contraceptives, anticonvulsants like gabapentin, corticosteroids like pred-nisone and even prescription-strength ibuprofen. This is even more alarming when we consider that some of these drugs are available over the counter.

Heart Sick: Heart Disease and Depression

Heart disease, one of the biggest killers worldwide, frequently occurs with depression—a tight connection that dissolves the barrier between mind and body. For serious cardiac issues, open-heart surgery falls firmly in the category where the benefit of surgery warrants the risk. But for less serious cardiac situations, we need to consider the relationship between heart health and depression. For decades, cardiac surgeons have acknowledged that depression is a comorbidity of open-heart surgery. This would not have surprised the ancient Dr. One, since each organ has its own emotional spirit in Chinese medicine. The heart's emotion is joy, and open-heart surgery directly disrupts the heart, the seat of joy.

While different strategies are employed to prevent depression in cardiac surgery suites, it remains a significant problem. And not only after heart surgery. People with depression often display impaired cardiovascular health, partially attributable to dysregulation of the autonomic nervous system and the higher incidence of inflammation.[12] The correlation with inflammatory markers is so significant that depression is now considered an inflammatory illness.

A Sinister Systems Synergy: Inflammation's Silent Song

In Chapter 6, we saw that the worse the autonomic balance, the greater the inflammation. With depression, we see poor autonomic balance leading to increased inflammation, which could not only play a role in causing depression but also lead to coronary artery disease.

Inflammation is closely associated with dysfunction in the endothelial lining of blood vessels, a precursor to atherosclerosis and atherothrombosis. Endothelial dysfunction has been detected in depression, and may prove to be a trait marker for the illness. Since higher rates of depression can lead to poor compliance with medications and treatment for cardiac disease, it can also lead to worse cardiac outcomes, even death. This sequence creates another vicious cycle, with our spiral going in the wrong direction and leading to the ultimate spiraling out of control.[13] Some researchers recommend using measures such as heart rate variability (HRV) to help screen and track this dysautonomia in depression.

A System Out of Balance: Autonomic Balance and Depression

Drug treatment with SSRIs might help with mood, but it does *not* address the autonomic imbalance. In a devilish observation, elevated levels of inflammation in patients with depression can lead to more frequent relapses.[14] Wait, what? How could this possibly be? Relapses, after all, must be related to the chemical imbalance, no? If not a chemical imbalance, what can explain the relapses?

The propensity for relapse may very well be due to *less innate resilience.* Remember, we saw that the better the HRV, a measure of flexibility and responsiveness, the more resilient the patient is. We also saw that autonomic balance and HRV correlate inversely with inflammatory markers, meaning the poorer the HRV, the higher the inflammatory markers. Increased levels of inflammation mean that the patient has a lower HRV and lower resilience to triggers and setbacks, and this makes them more likely to relapse.

Researchers like Dr. Kevin Tracey in the world of neuro-modulation have taken notice of this phenomenon, using implanted vagus nerve stimulation for major, treatment-resistant depression in hopes of helping restore autonomic balance.[15] Predictably, the results are mixed since man is not a machine. Still, these efforts may lead the way for hopeful new therapies.

Gut Punch: Depression and Inflammatory Bowel Disease

Inflammatory bowel disease also has depression as a comorbidity.[16] As noted, inflammatory bowel disease and depression are characterized by increases in proinflammatory cytokines TNF, Il-1β and Il-6 but lower levels of the anti-inflammatory cytokine Il-10.[17] Patients with depression and those with inflammatory bowel disease share this cytokine profile. Likewise, patients with inflammatory bowel disease have higher rates of depression, which illustrates Dr. One's principle that it all spins together.

In addition to therapies that directly affect autonomic balance, what about targeting brain inflammation itself as a treatment mode? Can we treat brain and mood conditions by treating inflammation in the body? To do that, we must reject and rethink our insistence on mind-body separation.

The Inflamed Mind: Inflammation and Brain Health

Professor Edward Bullmore, head of the department of psychiatry at Cambridge University author of *The Inflamed Mind*, says that low-grade inflammation, detectable only by blood tests, is increasingly considered part of the reason why common life experiences such as poverty, stress, obesity or aging are bad for public health.

As he wrote in *The Guardian*, "The reasonably well-informed hope—and I emphasize those words at this stage—is that targeting brain inflammation could lead to breakthroughs in *prevention* and treatment of depression, dementia, and psychosis on a par with the proven impact of immunological medicines for arthritis, cancer, and MS."[18] Professor Bullmore went on to point out that a drug initially licensed for multiple sclerosis was already being tried as a possible immune treatment for schizophrenia, and that results from many studies confirmed that bodily inflammation could cause changes in how the brain works. The philosophical prejudice against viewing the mind and body as deeply intertwined has segregated physical and mental health services, but Bullmore is hopeful that change is coming. He said, "The barrier between mind and body, for so long a dogmatic conviction, appears to be crumbling."

Of course, the distinction between mind and body never existed for Dr. One, so this would not have been news to him. All these systems are interrelated. We could say they all come down to inflammation, but looking further, we might even say they all come down to autonomic dysfunction. In some cases, stress is the cause. Stress causes hypervigilance, leading to an overabundance of sympathetic activity and less parasympathetic activity. We can't ignore the genetic component of depression (anterior heaven), but many cases of depression are not major or hereditary, and these cases might very well be appropriate for Dr. One and his gentle, gradual techniques. Suppose we could avoid a fraction of the suffering caused by depression and Dr. Two's repeated prescriptions for antidepressants, as in Laura's situation? We need to seriously consider the principle of doing no harm.

Remember, avoiding the bad is often more powerful than seeking the good. Suppose we employed Dr. One's strategies to increase vagal activity through, for example, yoga, meditation, breathing and acupuncture. By doing so, we would activate the macrophages, which stops the release of inflammatory cytokines such as TNF, Il-6 and Il-1B. Decreasing their inflammatory burden would help with depression and lessen inflammation in the coronary arteries. In patients with rheumatoid arthritis and inflammatory bowel disease, their disease burden would go down, and their associated depression would likely lighten. With the lightening of depression, motivation for healthy practices would improve, and the flywheel would be set into motion—all of which leads us to radical prevention.

Positive Systems Synergy for Resilience and Radical Prevention

Let's also remember that acupuncture points such as Stomach 36 increase parasympathetic activity. This can be another radical prevention strategy, as we saw in Chapter 6 with the studies on beagles and horses. When the beagles and horses were given acupuncture before a "startle" challenge, they had less autonomic reaction compared to control animals. We also saw how exposure to old friends, a hormetic stressor, helped to dampen an inflammatory response in the face of a mental stressor with the farmers versus the city dwellers in Chapter 6.

But also remember the study on student athletes discussed in Chapter 3, where acupuncture before a competitive event improved both cognitive anxiety and physiological autonomic markers of anxiety *preventatively.* While this benefited the athletes on the day of the meet, it might have also limited the negative flywheel effect of heightened vigilance and hidden inflammation.

This study and the other animal studies provide critical clues as to how Dr. One's techniques have the potential to be so effective. The first is that by giving the hormetic of acupuncture before a stressor, the body has more vagal activity and higher heart rate variability (HRV), which makes it is more resilient and more likely to brush off the event and resume homeostasis. The second implication of these studies is that by avoiding adverse autonomic reactions, the subjects also avoid negative health effects to their inflammatory profile, which can have far-reaching benefits. The third and equally important implication, though trickier to prove, is that the athletes may have set themselves up to avoid needing medications down the road.

When you consider this student-athlete study in the light of Laura's story, who was an overachieving student-athlete and scholar, ongoing performance stress may have been the genesis of her autonomic dysfunction. This could have led to inflammation and her depression. Perhaps an ounce of prevention would have been worth a pound of cure.

In Chapter 3, we heard the story of Teresa, who shed her panic attacks and became more functional with consistent acupuncture. By measuring her HRV during treatment, I could see it improve with acupuncture. Still, it's the clinical result that matters most, and it seemed that acupuncture also improved her susceptibility to panic attacks. After some treatment sessions, she could drive over bridges without triggering a panic attack. Who knows what would have happened if she had sought anti-anxiety medication instead? These sorts of hypothetical questions are worth asking, as we must carefully assess risk when considering which treatment options will keep the flywheel spinning. After all, the flywheel can go in two directions. We aim to keep it going in a positive one.

Resilience: A Buffer in the Face of Trouble

We have the physiological data to support the preventative effect of acupuncture. Without this data, the effects of acupuncture would most likely be explained away, as they repeatedly have been in the past, as a placebo and wishful thinking. That HRV is considered a marker for depression and correlates with cytokine load is a significant development. HRV can capture the autonomic activity over a period of seconds to minutes and over weeks to months.

But what really is HRV? It measures our favorite feedback, the autonomic nervous system, and how responsive and flexible it is. We know HRV decreases with stress, illness and old age. When 10- to 12-year-olds show lower HRV and they are highly socially anxious, their lower HRV can be a measure of their anxiety. But we now know that dampened HRV can have broader implications for the subsequent health of these children as well.[19] When HRV is depressed in teens, it can leave them less able to "roll with the punches" and more susceptible to anxiety disorders and mental distress. Improving HRV, autonomic balance and resilience could stave off depression, heart issues and maybe even inflammatory bowel disease. Doing all those things also has the considerable benefit of decreasing mental anguish, which is already epidemic in teens.

A broad study looking at women with depression noted that those with healthier HRV were less likely to spin out of control emotionally.[20] The authors call this the "dampening" or "buffering" effect of high HRV on the regulation difficulties of these at-risk women. Another study compared acupuncture and Prozac and found that acupuncture produced faster effects on mood.[21] Considering these results, the suggestion of seeking acupuncture for depression becomes much more bio-plausible and reasonable.

Depression and How "It All Spins Together"

With depression, we clearly see the potential of maintaining Dr. One's laws of maintaining balance by doing no harm. Remembering the example of the student athletes, and with autonomic balance as a measure, we see that we can maintain balance with acupuncture or other measures such as breathing, yoga or meditation. Strengthening our autonomic nervous system leads to less inflammation, a prime driver of depression and some of its comorbidities, such as heart disease. If we were to find ways to gently nudge the system of 10- to 12-year-olds with "old friends," acupuncture or breathing techniques, they might avoid the misery of social anxiety disorders.[22]

With depression, we see the mind-body connection as the tenuous separation that *the ancients never made*. Modern science is now catching up. The correlation between depression and cardiovascular disease, for example, has become too pronounced for the academic community to ignore. We've seen the latest science proving the interconnection of stress and poor autonomic balance, leading to increased inflammation. This runaway inflammation can manifest as heart disease, arthritis, inflammatory bowel disease and even depression.

In this stunning interplay, we witness the elegance of Dr. One's suggestion to avoid harm, engage in healthy practices, and receive treatments like acupuncture to regain balance. Gaining balance leads to more resilience and toughness in the face of adversity and may prevent spiraling out of control in various health issues. Once again, it all spins together in the synergy of our systems.

Chapter 9
Shooting for the Moon: Long Life, Great Health and New Strategies to Achieve Them

"Shoot for the moon. Even if you miss, you'll
land among the stars."
–Les Brown

Small Adjustments: The Wobbly Table Metaphor

The ancient Chinese parable of the table leg serves to distinguish the difference between ancient medicine and modern medicine. It goes like this: a table with one leg that is too long becomes wobbly and fragile. The carpenter equivalent of Dr. One would carefully turn the table over, sand the offending leg, turn the table back upright and check for stability. If the offending leg was still too long, he would repeat the procedure, painstakingly adjusting and honing the leg little by little until stability reigned.

The alternative approach would be to cut a portion off the long leg. This is quicker and easier, but carries the risk of over-cutting. If too much gets cut, the carpenter then has to shorten the other legs, and the table loses height. And this more drastic and expensive undertaking would still require adjustment and sanding afterward. Finally, ignoring the wobbly table from the get-go and doing nothing can lead to greater instability, more extensive repairs or the need to throw out the table altogether.

The message of the analogy is simple: taking care of a minor imbalance before it requires a more comprehensive repair, such as replacing the entire leg or throwing the table away, is better. Since we only have one body, it's best to treat it with care since we don't have the luxury of throwing it out and starting over.

We are lucky to live in a time when we have the means to take dramatic action in the face of severe "broken legs." Modern medicine has been miraculous with breakthroughs in gene therapy, prosthetics, insulin, L-DOPA, deep brain stimulation, trauma centers, ICU facilities and prenatal care—the list is endless. But we've seen that even the big killers are susceptible to Dr. One's methods.

Because inflammation is so tightly connected to autonomic and vagal activity, we can lower inflammation by increasing vagal activity and decreasing sympathetic activity. In doing so, we can hopefully avoid drastic and often risky measures and stay in a place of safety, where we've done no harm.

Follow the Science

In the context of systems biology and complexity tools such as heart rate variability (HRV), we can provide quantitative evidence for once-vague concepts such as wellness or well-being. We can now measure inflammatory messengers, making the invisible inflammation visible. I hope to help shift the model from *man-as-machine* to *man-as-homeostatic-system-seeking-balance*. While this description doesn't roll off the tongue, it is more accurate. This model allows for self-healing, using minor stressors and avoiding harm to stay in balance. But more than that, it allows for a whole new concept of the possible.

The aspirational possibility of "radical resilience," becomes imaginable where a person can become sturdier and tougher through treatment and practices to better withstand life's various challenges. When we can accept that certain measures will improve our "posterior heaven" (our "epigenetics"), we improve our odds of achieving a long and robust life, and of "getting an edge." This vision is the "moonshot" I mentioned in Chapter One and it is based firmly on the pillar of Dr. One's methods: balance.

A final metaphor for this balance is seeking strategies that provide "ballast" for your system—a deep stability so that you don't rock wildly out of control or capsize when turbulence occurs. The role of the vagus nerve in engendering this stability appears throughout the book. Autonomic balance and the vagus nerve link everything together—immunity, mood, pain, longevity and beyond. There may be other safe ways to engender this balance besides maintaining autonomic balance that have not yet been discovered. But we need to be *open* to recognizing them to find them. We must keep our minds receptive and our models *fluid*. This open-mindedness will help advance the moonshot mission.

Three Ways to Think About Alternative Therapies

Before our final moon landing, there are good reasons to adopt at least some of the alternative strategies mentioned in this book:

1. **Keep safety in mind.** Investigating, refining and employing non-invasive therapies is typically very low risk.
2. **Even if the results aren't definitive in one area, they can benefit the person as a whole since *our systems are in synergy and it all spins together*.** For example, better sleep leads to

better mood and less pain and can set up a positive feedback loop in the right direction.

3. **See the "bigger picture" of alternative therapies.** Although some alternatives are relatively expensive to the patient since they are often not covered by insurance, they are economical overall by promising better health and less risk with fewer interventions and medications.

Of course, we are not there yet. I confront the limitations of balancing strategies daily in my practice. We are a long way from being able to quantify and personalize these gentle but powerful treatments decisively and systematically. I have an advantage in that I've seen first-hand, time and time again, remarkable results for patients—sometimes incrementally and sometimes all at once. I'm also heartened when I reflect on how much the scientific community has learned over a relatively short time, that is just since I've been in practice. As research proves acupuncture's benefits, it motivates me and gives me hope.

Modern Science Validates Acupuncture's Effects

We've gone from acupuncture effects being attributed to gating or dismissed as a placebo to having acupuncture's impact confirmed by high-profile scientists through the healing power of the vagus nerve. More recently, through the mind-bending capabilities of modern science, we have found a way to remotely stimulate nerves with light (optogenetic nerve stimulation) to reveal some peripheral nerves as more potent vagal stimulators than others (as mentioned in Chapter 6). This single discovery not only validates those of us studying acupuncture's effect on vagal activity, but also shows that different acupuncture points have different effects. This mainstay of ancient practice was never scientifically verified until recently and could have enormous implications.

But using optogenetic nerve stimulation instead of needling also underscores the potential for entirely novel ways to stimulate acupuncture points that might make acupuncture more accessible, cheaper, and perhaps even allow remote delivery systems. A recent study (albeit a pilot, small bore study) used LED light stimulation on two commonly used acupuncture points and could compare the effect of the two points stimulated at different frequencies on the subject's heart rate variability (HRV).[1] This kind of treatment would obviate needling and could even lead to home-based treatment, making acupuncture more convenient.

These and other discoveries invite novel approaches to acupuncture treatment to make it more effective. It could also validate personalized treatment, another pillar of ancient teachings. But acupuncture aside, there could be ramifications for many branches of medicine and health practices.

A significant caveat: all of the studies I've cited in this book need rigorous testing, a practice woefully absent in medical research. A striking example is the specter of doubt being raised about Alzheimer's research landmark studies that show how flimsy even famous research commanding massive amounts of grant money can be. Remember John Oliver's remark about replication studies, that there are no Nobel Prizes for fact-checking. We also know that there are intense incentives to publish. But just the fact that we have acupuncture research that can be put under the microscope is a testament to how far we've come.

One Area of Medicine Affects Others: Research Synergy

The story of this book comes down to witnessing scientific discovery in real time and my urge to share it. My exploration started with the question of how acupuncture could have affected my allergies, launching a meandering journey of inquiry, research and documentation. It's a process that started from a narrow focus on acupuncture which, by necessity, broadened to immunology, brain regions, mechanics of inflammation, the autonomic nervous system and beyond. Whole swaths of medicine became relevant to my question.

Following this question, it became apparent how one area of medicine affects others. Powerful computer modeling could explain the most subtle physiological systems, from brain imaging to autonomic monitoring. Advances in biochemistry led to the ability to measure microscopic quantities of inflammatory and immune markers. A discovery in one field affected unrelated ones, sometimes incrementally and sometimes all at once with seemingly miraculous breakthroughs.

Expanding Your Mental Models: Be Willing to Give Alternatives a Try

A critical task in telling this story was introducing an alternative medical approach, which required a shift in mental models. Because I had two potent life experiences, my stressful time in Switzerland and the dramatic acupuncture "crisis of cure" with my allergies, I was more willing to entertain alternative medical models despite my decades of Western medical experience and training. I like to think that introducing these alternative medical models is easier now because we have more evidence. And I also want to think that having this scientific underpinning gives "permission" to patients to try alternative approaches who otherwise wouldn't consider it.

In my practice, when I give patients this "permission" to leave a medication behind, it allows them to take some time to consider options other than what traditional medicine advises. Because I'm a medical doctor, perhaps they find it easier to consider alternatives. Rita Redberg, an editor for JAMA and cardiology expert at UCSF, also sees this validation as an important function she fulfills. Patients fly across the country to consult with her, often getting permission to stop their statins, bone density tests or radiology scans.

Shooting for the Moon

There could be a long way to go; getting to the moon is a long shot, after all. But I am guardedly optimistic. Medical research has its own interlocking systems of study that feed on each other with its own systems synergy. The tedious, focused, incremental research in many fields suddenly converges overnight into a quantum shift. And we can only guess what further advances we might encounter, any one of which might enable a breakthrough for our moon landing. Please read on for strategies and practices that can help you on your journey to balance, resilience and a longer life.

Chapter 10
Stoking the Flywheel: Small Steps, Big Results and the Power Law of Systems Synergy

"The doctor of the future will give no medicine but will interest his patients in the care of the human frame, in diet and in the cause and prevention of disease."
–Thomas Edison

How can you use the science and ancient wisdom you've learned in this book and make them part of your everyday life? Remember our discussion of anterior and posterior heaven? While you can't do much about your anterior heaven (your genetics or what you are born with), you can improve your posterior heaven (your environment and lifestyle). Improving some of your habits and choices under your control can help engender resilience, toughness and a longer life.

We have learned that Dr. One strives for balance which he nurtures with hormetics, small challenges which make us tougher. We have the powerful image of the flywheel, where we develop momentum that takes us beyond simple safety to a place where positive feedback loops are in motion to create even better health, mood and longevity. Unfortunately, there is no ratchet system for this flywheel (like we have in cable cars in my native San Francisco). We can backslide as well. But as James Clear points out in *Atomic Habits*, small habits or interventions don't just add up; they compound.[1] Acupuncture can be a powerful impetus in the right direction, but the principle of hormesis pertains even if you have no access to acupuncture.

I appreciate that standing at the bottom of a giant mountain of potential change can seem daunting, if not impossible. You might even question *Why try?* One approach is to consider incorporating the strategies that most appeal to you. You don't have to do them all. Remember, in systems biology, small inputs can lead to substantial results: the essence of nonlinearity. Each system affects the others, and consistency is more powerful than intensity when it comes to habits. A hormetic challenge is like slowly sanding and not sawing the table leg. Accepting the possibility of nonlinearity and the potential for more significant changes can turn any thoughts of defeatism upside down. Change can happen incrementally, but sometimes it comes in quantum leaps.

We *can* improve our sleep with some tweaks. We *can* add modest amounts of exercise. We *can* put off eating breakfast for a few minutes. We *can* breathe deeply. We *can* make some acupuncture appointments. And it all spins together. You can see differences beyond what you imagine by instituting small changes and turning them into habits. You can slowly (or quickly!) develop the deep strength necessary to take toxins, accidents, heartbreak and sudden stressors in stride—and live long by doing so.

The Multiple Benefits of Exercise

Exercise provides multiple health benefits, of course. It strengthens the heart, improves sleep, is a potent anti-inflammatory strategy and slows cognitive decline. You don't have to run a marathon or a four-minute mile to see these benefits. Various studies have shown such benefits when doing far less:

- One study showed that aerobic exercise 150 minutes a week (the equivalent of five 30-minute sessions) helps slow cognitive decline.[2]
- Moderate exercise once a week and other modest lifestyle changes reduced cardiac deaths in elderly patients by 46 percent.[3]
- Moderate intensity endurance training for 30 to 40 minutes, five days a week, improved BP, lipid tolerance and glucose regulation.[4]

Even minimal amounts of exercise can reap rewards. Prominent acupuncture researcher Luis Ulloa found that after putting mice through just *one session* of moderate exercise, they had a decrease in inflammatory cytokines(including tumor necrosis factor (TNF)) and an increase in anti-inflammatory cytokines. He also found a lowered tumor necrosis factor and an increase in dopamine via vagus nerve activity.[5] The consensus is that no matter how much exercise you do, don't skip more than two days if you can help it.

Sauna

If you can get access to a sauna, use it. And use it as often as you can because you may well experience numerous health advantages. The sauna is a classic hormetic challenge: it stresses your body in a limited way, triggering your thermoregulatory systems so they are alert and robust.

Studies conducted by Finnish researcher J. A. Laukkanen show that taking a sauna four to seven times a week for at least 20 minutes a session at 174 degrees Fahrenheit provides a robust reduction in memory loss, illness and all-cause mortality.[6] Heat causes a decrease of toxic protein aggregates associated with neurodegenerative diseases such as Alzheimer's, Parkinson's and Huntington's disease.

Sauna use lowers inflammatory markers such as C-reactive protein and fibrinogen and positively modulates total cholesterol, low-density lipoprotein cholesterol, high-density lipoprotein cholesterol and triglycerides. There is also evidence that sauna exposure could boost the immune system, partly explaining the reduced susceptibility to common colds and prevention of infections in healthy individuals who sauna regularly.

Additionally, sauna use also decreases cardiac disease deaths and improves cardiac risk profile. Its anti-inflammatory effects, which reduce the risk of neurodegenerative diseases and improve cardiac health, most likely contribute to overall longevity improvement.

Most saunas are of the Finnish type, hot and dry. Infrared saunas have become popular but are not as hot, so you may need to lengthen your sessions for optimal response.

Cold Exposure

It's crucial that cold exposure, just like heat exposure, is at a hormetic dose—challenging but not extreme. It can help you live longer. As longevity expert Dr. David Sinclair says, "Exposing your body to less-than-comfortable temperatures is another very effective way to turn on your longevity genes."[7] Colder temperatures do this through their ability to rev up brown adipose tissue, though cold and exercise together build brown fat even more.[8] Brown fat breaks down blood sugar (glucose) and fat molecules to create heat and help maintain body temperature.

So, how do you get colder? It can be anything from taking cold showers to leaving a window open at night, or even something as simple as using a lighter blanket. Swimming in chilly water is another excellent option for those who find it exhilarating or at least tolerable! If you are intrigued by this strategy, the multi-pronged approach of Dutchman Wim Hof, famous for his ability to withstand extreme cold and nicknamed The Iceman, might be a valuable resource.[9]

Diet

I'm reluctant to weigh in on diet since it is such a vast and personal topic. Many of us have watched diets come and go, bewildered by how some foods we thought were healthy are now shunned and vice versa. Even so, the Mediterranean diet is an excellent place to start as it is sustainable and delicious. It is the opposite of a fad diet since it has been around for millennia.

The diet prioritizes:

- Whole grains, fruits, vegetables, legumes, nuts, herbs, spices and olive oil.
- Fish rich in Omega-3 fatty acids like salmon, sardines and tuna as being the preferred source of animal proteins.
- Chicken or turkey, eaten sparingly.
- Foods high in saturated fats, like red meat and butter, eaten rarely.
- Eggs and dairy products like yogurt and cheese, eaten in moderation.

These guidelines lead to better health and particularly better heart health. The Mediterranean diet has been shown to help lower blood sugar, reduce inflammation and lower body mass index. It also protects against oxidative stress, which can lead to neurological disease and cancer. One feature of the Mediterranean diet is that it is rich in fiber, which can lead to a healthy microbiome.

With this advice, we need to keep in mind that each

person is different. Each person's needs vary at different times of their lives, so "healthy" diets can vary as well.

Time-Restricted Eating and Fasting

Intermittent fasting is an excellent hormetic challenge, causing cells to "hunker down" and increase autophagy (getting rid of old cells), which helps with inflammation and can turn on the cellular mechanisms leading to longevity, such as lower levels of IGF-1.

"Fasting as part of daily life and longevity seem to go hand in hand," says longevity expert Dr. David Sinclair, giving the example of the Greek island of Ikaria where religious fasting is a frequent occurrence and a third of the population lives beyond 90.[10] Similarly, in Bama County, China, another locus of longevity, many of its centenarians skip breakfast, eat a small meal at noon and a larger meal with family at twilight.

Such time-restricted eating is an alternative to intermittent or outright fasting. One suggested regimen is fasting for 15 or 16 hours straight per day. Another option is to eat 75 percent fewer calories two days a week. While attractive for weight loss, the more significant benefit is overall health with decreased inflammation leading to improved longevity. If you choose to go the route of plain calorie restriction (not fun!), there is evidence it helps with cognitive decline.[11]

Nutritional Supplements

The FDA estimates there are more than 29,000 different supplements in the marketplace and an average of 1,000 new products each year.[12] Keep in mind that the FDA must approve medicines *before* they can be sold or marketed, but supplements do not require this approval. I will share a few nutritional supplements here, along with their perceived benefits.

Coenzyme Q10: There is evidence that the antioxidant effect of CoQ10 alleviates cardiovascular disease and inflammation (remember, though, that antioxidants may have some negative effects). Coenzyme Q levels have been found to be lower in people with dementia.[13]

L-Serine: The amino acid L-serine can counter the effects of a toxin that causes neurodegenerative disease. It is also a focus of intense research as a possible mitigator of Alzheimer's. It is inexpensive and safe.[14]

NMN: As we age, our levels of nicotinamide adenine dinucleotide (NAD+), an alternative form of the B3 vitamin, plummet dramatically. Dr. David Sinclair, the longevity expert, recommends supplementation with nicotinamide mononucleotide (NMN). NMN supplementation reportedly increased NAD+ biosynthesis, suppressed age-related adipose tissue inflammation, enhanced insulin secretion and action, improved mitochondrial function and improved neuronal function in the brain.

The FDA recently advised against taking NMN, but is not banning it from the marketplace.[15] This confusing state of affairs leaves the decision of whether to take it or not in limbo. I include this here since it is relevant to Dr. Sinclair's work and may end up becoming a valuable supplement for longevity.

Astragalus: The herb astragalus is a mainstay of Chinese medicine. Studies show it improves telomere length, which correlates with longevity.[16] Traditionally, it is used in conjunction with other herbs as an overall tonic to stay well and live long.

Vitamin D: "Vitamin D is crucial for control of about five percent of the human genome," says Rhonda Patrick,

Ph.D.[17] Low vitamin D levels have been associated with increased aging, all-cause mortality and the likelihood of testing positive for COVID-19 during the pandemic. Vitamin D is important for DNA repair and anti-inflammatory substances, both of which are responsible for telomere length. A large multi-country study showed that Vitamin D cut infection risk by 50 percent. In post-menopausal women, vitamin D increased muscle strength by 25 percent.[18] Low heart rate variability (HRV), a sign of age, stress and disease, correlates with lower levels of vitamin D in the blood. What's the recommended amount you should take each day? Dr. Patrick says 4000 IU.

Probiotics: There is a rich body of research on the role of our gut bacteria on our immunity, mental health and overall resilience. Our friend, the vagus nerve, plays a crucial role in the interface between the gut, brain and immune system. One of the levers triggering the vagus nerve is our microbiome, the billions of bacteria living in our gut. A diverse microbiome is a crucial feature of a healthy gastrointestinal system, but diversity can be lacking in patients with depression, the elderly, anyone recently traumatized physically or mentally or anyone who recently took antibiotics.

I will limit the discussion of microbiomes here since so many books have been written on the topic, but I recommend that you take a probiotic to cover your bases. Products are available that won't break the bank, and they may be one more nudge to help keep your flywheel spinning. Be sure to include foods in your diet with plenty of fiber, as a fiber-rich diet encourages diversity of the microbiome, too.

Prebiotics: Consider incorporating prebiotics or forms of fermented food in your diet. According to recent research, fermented foods like kimchee, sauerkraut, buttermilk and yogurt can improve the diversity of your microbiome. Elie

Metchnikoff, a founder of the field of immunology discussed in Chapter 5, noticed over 100 years ago that a subpopulation in Bulgaria was living longer. He surmised that it was due to eating a lot of fermented milk products. His observation caused a craze of yogurt consumption that has continued to this day.

Sleep

Sleep expert Matthew Walker has written over 100 research papers on sleep. His best-selling book, *Why We Sleep: Unlocking the Power of Sleep and Dreams,* shares some compelling reasons why we need to sleep to improve our well-being.[19] Consider the following for improved sleep:

Light: Light can be key depending on when and how you get it. Ideally, you want to get sunlight soon after waking up. According to Stanford neurologist Andrew Huberman, if you rise before dawn, you should turn on strong overhead lights, which hit the part of your eye that is most effective at getting the beneficial effects of light in the morning.[20] Bright light helps to suppress your melatonin and wake you up. During the day, work with natural light if possible and get sunlight at twilight. Light during the day helps trigger your melatonin, a hormone that enables sleep. Before bed, avoid bright screen light from computers, tablets and cell phones. Even avoid other lights in the bedroom, such as a digital clock.

Temperature: You need your body temperature to drop so you can sleep well, so keep your room cool. Consider using fewer blankets. A hot bath before bed can relax your muscles and reset your thermostat to counteract the heat so that you cool down for sleeping.

Beds are for sleeping: If you wake up in the middle of the night and can't get back to sleep, it's best to get up and go to another room. Take some analog reading material, not a screen, but make sure it's not a page-turner you won't be able to put down! Once you start getting sleepy, return to bed. Try to avoid checking the time.

Caffeine and alcohol: Avoid caffeine for eight hours before going to bed. Caffeine can stay in your system for a long time and disrupt your deep, non-REM sleep. Sleep researchers shun caffeine altogether because they are convinced of its harmful effects, and sleep expert Dr. Matthew Walker recommends others do the same.[21] Similarly, don't consume alcohol close to bedtime, as it can interfere with your REM sleep and leave you more tired overall.

Take a Deep Breath

Bestselling author Dr. Andrew Weil recommends a simple breathing exercise for anxiety or stress, which you can also use before sleep or if you wake up at night.[22] It seems to lower blood pressure and improve digestion and mood, probably from vagal increase and lower sympathetic outflow (fight-or-flight). Here's how to do it:

- Exhale completely through your mouth, making a *whoosh* sound.
- Close your mouth and inhale quietly through your nose to a mental count of four.
- Hold your breath for a count of seven.
- Exhale completely through your mouth, making a *whoosh* sound to a count of eight.
- Do this exercise four times twice a day for four to six weeks. After that, you can increase it to eight times twice a day.

Another breathing approach is "box breathing," a simple technique taught to Navy SEALs to help calm fight-or-flight. Use this technique in times of stress or if you wake up in the middle of the night to help you fall back asleep. It increases vagal activity and requires a bit of thought, which can help distract an overactive brain. Here's what to do:

- Picture a square box to help guide your breathing; imagine the sides of the box represent inhale, hold, exhale and hold, each step taking four seconds.
- Breathe in for four seconds and hold for four seconds.
- Breathe out for four seconds and hold for four seconds.
- Do this for three to four minutes.

If you want a more specific practice, Andrew Huberman recommends measuring your carbon dioxide release time and then using that number for the number of seconds on each side of the box. He stresses that nasal breathing is best on inhalation because it allows you to fill your lungs better.

Huberman also published a paper showing that box breathing, hyperventilation and cyclic sighing all improved mood when practiced five minutes a day for a month.[23] These breathing practices were all superior to meditation. The best was cyclic sighing, a technique where you perform a big inhale, then another smaller one filling your lungs as much as possible through your nose and then releasing all air through your mouth. The goal is to improve your breathing by counteracting the tendency to breathe too quickly. This breath training helps make the breathing dynamics better.

Wim Hof has designed a more intense breathing regimen that confers many health benefits as well.[24]

Herbal Therapy

Herbal therapy is a vast subject and is not covered in this book. There are plenty of practitioners who incorporate Chinese herbal formulas with every patient. I use herbs also, but it is not the mainstay of my practice. However, I prescribe herbs when the risk-to-benefit calculation warrants it.

Acupuncture

Acupuncture is a huge topic in and of itself, filling entire libraries. As you have read, my area of interest is the interface of acupuncture and autonomic balance and measuring it with heart rate variability (HRV). This fascination and focus is my small niche and unique to my practice. Little did I know when I started focusing on autonomic balance and vagal activity that it would be a critical fulcrum for so many health conditions. What follows are the basic considerations for acupuncture treatment. There is a range of practitioners, and some might be a better fit for you than others.

Medical Acupuncture versus "Lay" Acupuncture

I am a "medical acupuncturist," a Western-trained physician practicing acupuncture. Because I spent my medical career in anesthesiology, a specialty heavily reliant on learning and mastering physiological measurements, I have a keen interest in physiological monitoring. I'm interested in academic medical research in general because I can't help but think it will improve my results.

There are advantages for patients who seek out medical acupuncture because of the extensive training needed to become a physician. But most lay acupuncturists also provide excellent care and have deep knowledge. In seeking a practitioner, I recommend the usual due diligence of asking around, reading reviews and interviewing prospective acupuncturists. But one of the most important things is to find someone in close proximity to you, as it is crucial to keep appointments.

Treatment and Timing

Typically, two sessions per week or more are optimal when starting treatment for a chronic condition, followed by weekly treatment. Some of my patients continue to come in weekly because they see the benefit. But many others come in monthly or quarterly, which can also work to keep symptoms at bay.

Associated Treatments in Conjunction with Acupuncture

Ear Tacks

Ear tacks are tiny needles on a small, unobtrusive piece of tape that the patient can wear for up to two weeks before changing them. They are helpful for many conditions but seem particularly useful for sleeping, anxiety, blood pressure and digestion. The patient can remove them and they are safe. Ear seeds are an alternative to ear tacks, but I use tacks because I think the slight injury they invoke is advantageous.

Transcutaneous Auricular Vagal Nerve Stimulation (TAVNS)

Transcutaneous Auricular Vagal Stimulation (TAVNS) is another way to increase vagal activity, at least theoretically. It is the subject of a great deal of research and uses noninvasive stimulation on the ear.

The ear has innervation from the auricular branch of the

vagus nerve. It is thought that stimulating this nerve will increase vagal activity throughout the body. It is popular with some patients. The hope is that it will provide reinforcing treatment patients can apply at home. Studies are underway on this therapy around the globe. Because TAVNS fits my criteria for safety, I'm exploring it in conjunction with HRV and acupuncture, of course!

———

By using the strategies shared above in your daily life, you will see and feel a difference. Some of them may compound so that you see changes and feel better gradually or all at once, which is the essence of nonlinearity.

Another dictum of Chinese medicine is that humans live between heaven and earth. We look to the heavens for inspiration, air and the mysteries of the unseen. But our feet are on the ground—solid, textured and part of us. Yet we are also of the sea, as we are more than half water. We are none of these —not sky, earth or water. But at the same time, we are all three. We are born "nonlinear" and part of nature itself. We share the fractal beauty of a fern, the clouds, the shoreline or the breakers. Our bodies and minds are part of nature, built with feedback loops and systems to be balanced, challenged and coaxed along. This is the power and wisdom of Dr. One. Now that you know about it, play with it! Use it in good health on your way to radical resilience and live long!

Notes

1. In Search of Doctor One: Embracing Nature's Laws for Radical Prevention and Long Life

1. US Centers for Medicare & Medicaid Services (2021). *National Health Expenditure fact sheet.* https://www.cms.gov/research-statistics-data-and-systems/statistics-trends-and-reports/nationalhealthexpenddata/nhe-fact-sheet

2. John Hopkins Medicine. (2016, May 3). Study suggests medical errors now third leading cause of death in the US [press release]. https://www.hopkinsmedicine.org/news/media/releases/study_suggests_medical_errors_now_third_leading_cause_of_death_in_the_us

3. Gunja, M. Z., Gumas, E. D., & Williams, R. D. (2023). US health care from a global perspective, 2022: accelerating spending, worsening outcomes. *The Commonwealth Fund. Published January 21.*

4. Isaacson, W. (2011). *Steve Jobs.* Simon & Schuster. https://www.simonandschuster.com/books/Steve-Jobs/Walter-Isaacson/9781982176860

5. Harman, J. (2014). *The Shark's Paintbrush: Biomimicry and How Nature is Inspiring Innovation.* White Cloud Press.

6. Lancellotti, P., Marechal, P., Donis, N., & Oury, C. (2019). Inflammation, cardiovascular disease, and cancer: a common link with far-reaching implications. *European Heart Journal, 40*(48), 3910-3912.

7. https://www.brainyquote.com/quotes/henry_david_thoreau_705811

2. Do No Harm

1. Slusser, S. (2020, April 12). A's Gone By: Reliever Micah Bowie deals with harrowing lung problems. *San Francisco Chronicle.* https://www.sfchronicle.com/athletics/article/A-s-Gone-By-Reliever-Micah-Bowie-deals-with-15214077.php

2. Slusser, S. (2020, April 12). A's Gone By: Reliever Micah Bowie deals with harrowing lung problems. *San Francisco Chronicle.* https://www.sfchronicle.com/athletics/article/A-s-Gone-By-Reliever-Micah-Bowie-deals-with-15214077.php

3. Gracian, B. (2013). *The art of worldly wisdom.* Createspace Publishing. https://blas.com/the-art-of-worldly-wisdom/

4. https://quotefancy.com/quote/1561887/Charlie-Munger-All-I-want-to-know-is-where-I-m-going-to-die-so-I-ll-never-go-there

Notes

5. John Hopkins Medicine. (2016, May 3). Study suggests medical errors now third leading cause of death in the US [press release]. https://www.hopkinsmedicine.org/news/media/releases/study_suggests_medical_errors_now_third_leading_cause_of_death_in_the_us

6. Epstein, D. (2017, February 22). When evidence says no but doctors say yes. *ProPublica*. https://www.propublica.org/article/when-evidence-says-no-but-doctors-say-yes

7. Centers for Disease Control and Prevention. *Heart disease facts*. (2023, May 15). Retrieved May 15, 2023, from https://www.cdc.gov/heartdisease/facts.htm

8. Khera, A. V., Emdin, C. A., Drake, I., Natarajan, P., Bick, A. G., Cook, N. R., ... & Kathiresan, S. (2016). Genetic risk, adherence to a healthy lifestyle, and coronary disease. *New England Journal of Medicine, 375*(24), 2349-2358.

9. Edney, A. & Tracer, Z. (2016, November 28). Funding for cures bill remains sticking point for health groups. *Bloomberg*. https://www.bloomberg.com/news/articles/2016-11-28/funding-for-cures-bill-remains-sticking-point-for-health-groups

10. Katz, M. H., Grady, D., & Redberg, R. F. (2014). Developing methods for less is more. *JAMA internal medicine, 174*(7), 1076-1076.

11. Last Week Tonight. (2016, May 8). Scientific studies: last week tonight with John Oliver (HBO) [Video]. YouTube. https://www.youtube.com/watch?v=0Rnq1NpHdmw

12. https://www.propublica.org/article/when-evidence-says-no-but-doctors-say-yes

13. Epstein, D. (2017, February 22). When evidence says no but doctors say yes. *ProPublica*. https://www.propublica.org/article/when-evidence-says-no-but-doctors-say-yes

14. Allan, G. M., Spooner, G. R., & Ivers, N. (2012). X-ray scans for nonspecific low back pain: A nonspecific pain?. *Canadian Family Physician, 58*(3), 275-275.

15. Bovey, M. (2017, January 25). Rapid Response: Acupuncture: is NICE cutting off its nose to spite its face? *BMJ*. https://www.bmj.com/content/356/bmj.i6748/rr-7

3. Your Stress Response: The Deep Power of Balance

1. Sapolsky, R. M. (1994). *Why Zebras Don't Get Ulcers: An updated guide to stress, stress-related diseases, and coping*. W.H. Freeman and Company.

2. Sparrow, K. (2007). Analysis of heart rate variability in acupuncture practice: can it improve outcomes? *Medical Acupuncture, 19*(1), 37-42. https://www.liebertpub.com/doi/abs/10.1089/acu.2006.0000

3. Bäcker, M., Grossman, P., Schneider, J., Michalsen, A., Knoblauch, N., Tan, L., ... & Dobos, G. J. (2008). Acupuncture in migraine: investigation of autonomic effects. *The Clinical journal of pain, 24*(2), 106-115.

Notes

4. Maccariello, C. E. M., de Souza, C. C. F., Morena, L., Dias, D. P. M., & de Medeiros, M. A. (2018). Effects of acupuncture on the heart rate variability, cortisol levels and behavioural response induced by thunder sound in beagles. *Physiology & behavior, 186*, 37-44.

5. Villas-Boas, J. D., Dias, D. P. M., Trigo, P. I., Almeida, N. A. D. S., de Almeida, F. Q., & de Medeiros, M. A. (2015). Acupuncture affects autonomic and endocrine but not behavioural responses induced by startle in horses. *Evidence-Based Complementary and Alternative Medicine, 2015*.

6. Zarei, S., Shayestehfar, M., Memari, A. H., SeifBarghi, T., & Sobhani, V. (2017). Acupuncture decreases competitive anxiety prior to a competition in young athletes: a randomized controlled trial pilot study. *Journal of Complementary and Integrative Medicine, 14*(1), 20150085.

7. Sparrow, K., & Golianu, B. (2014). Does acupuncture reduce stress over time? A clinical heart rate variability study in hypertensive patients. *Medical acupuncture, 26*(5), 286-294.

8. Mehta, P. K., Polk, D. M., Zhang, X., Li, N., Painovich, J., Kothawade, K., ... & Merz, C. N. B. (2014). A randomized controlled trial of acupuncture in stable ischemic heart disease patients. *International journal of cardiology, 176*(2), 367-374.

9. Torres-Rosas, R., Yehia, G., Peña, G., Mishra, P., del Rocio Thompson-Bonilla, M., Moreno-Eutimio, M. A., ... & Ulloa, L. (2014). Dopamine mediates vagal modulation of the immune system by electroacupuncture. *Nature medicine, 20*(3), 291-295.

10. Gidron, Y., Deschepper, R., De Couck, M., Thayer, J. F., & Velkeniers, B. (2018). The vagus nerve can predict and possibly modulate non-communicable chronic diseases: introducing a neuroimmunological paradigm to public health. *Journal of clinical medicine, 7*(10), 371.

11. Ahn, A. C., Nahin, R. L., Calabrese, C., Folkman, S., Kimbrough, E., Shoham, J., & Haramati, A. (2010). Applying principles from complex systems to studying the efficacy of CAM therapies. *Journal of alternative and complementary medicine (New York, N.Y.), 16*(9), 1015–1022. https://doi.org/10.1089/acm.2009.0593.

12. Jarczok, M. N., Kleber, M. E., Koenig, J., Loerbroks, A., Herr, R. M., Hoffmann, K., ... & Thayer, J. F. (2015). Investigating the associations of self-rated health: heart rate variability is more strongly associated than inflammatory and other frequently used biomarkers in a cross sectional occupational sample. *PloS one, 10*(2), e0117196.

13. Paniccia, M., Paniccia, D., Thomas, S., Taha, T., & Reed, N. (2017). Clinical and non-clinical depression and anxiety in young people: A scoping review on heart rate variability. *Autonomic Neuroscience, 208*, 1-14.

14. Gidron, Y., Deschepper, R., De Couck, M., Thayer, J. F., & Velkeniers, B. (2018). The vagus nerve can predict and possibly modulate non-communicable chronic diseases: introducing a neuroimmunological paradigm to public health. *Journal of clinical medicine, 7*(10), 371.

4. Longevity: Unlocking Our Cells' Secrets to Defy Aging

1. Suwen, N. (1995). *The Yellow Emperor's Classic of Medicine* (M. Ni PhD, Trans.). Shambala.
2. Epel, E. S., Blackburn, E. H., Lin, J., Dhabhar, F. S., Adler, N. E., Morrow, J. D., & Cawthon, R. M. (2004). Accelerated telomere shortening in response to life stress. *Proceedings of the National Academy of Sciences, 101*(49), 17312-17315.
3. Wdowiak, A., Raczkiewicz, D., Janczyk, P., Bojar, I., Makara-Studzińska, M., & Wdowiak-Filip, A. (2020). Interactions of cortisol and prolactin with other selected menstrual cycle hormones affecting the chances of conception in infertile women. *International Journal of Environmental Research and Public Health, 17*(20), 7537.
4. Sinclair, D. & LaPlante, M.D. (2019). *Lifespan: why we age—and why we don't have to.* Atria Books.
5. Averill, G. (2019, November 9). This scientist believes aging is optional. Outside. https://www.outsideonline.com/health/wellness/lifespan-david-sinclair-book-review/
6. Tazearslan, C., Huang, J., Barzilai, N., & Suh, Y. (2011). Impaired IGF1R signaling in cells expressing longevity-associated human IGF1R alleles. *Aging cell, 10*(3), 551-554.
7. Gurinovich, A., Song, Z., Zhang, W., Federico, A., Monti, S., Andersen, S. L., ... & Sebastiani, P. (2021). Effect of longevity genetic variants on the molecular aging rate. *GeroScience, 43*(3), 1237-1251.
8. Petrick, H. L., King, T. J., Pignanelli, C., Vanderlinde, T. E., Cohen, J. N., Holloway, G. P., & Burr, J. F. (2021). Endurance and Sprint Training Improve Glycemia and V˙ O2peak but only Frequent Endurance Benefits Blood Pressure and Lipidemia. *Medicine and Science in Sports and Exercise, 53*(6), 1194-1205.
9. Laukkanen, J. A., Laukkanen, T., & Kunutsor, S. K. (2018, August). Cardiovascular and other health benefits of sauna bathing: a review of the evidence. In *Mayo clinic proceedings* (Vol. 93, No. 8, pp. 1111-1121). Elsevier.
10. Kulkarni, A. S., Gubbi, S., & Barzilai, N. (2020). Benefits of metformin in attenuating the hallmarks of aging. *Cell metabolism, 32*(1), 15-30.
11. Selvarani, R., Mohammed, S., & Richardson, A. (2021). Effect of rapamycin on aging and age-related diseases—past and future. *Geroscience, 43*, 1135-1158.
12. Velasquex-Manoff, M. (2014, June 25). *Fruits and vegetables are trying to kill you.* Nautilus. https://nautil.us/fruits-and-vegetables-are-trying-to-kill-you-2155/
13. Ball, P. "Yes, Life in the Fast Lane Kills You." *Nautilus.* May 2, 2016. https://getpocket.com/explore/item/yes-life-in-the-fast-lane-kills-you/
14. Lipsitz, L. (2016, May 20). *The real secret of youth is complexity.* Nautilus. Ahttps://nautil.us/the-real-secret-of-youth-is-complexity-235951/
15. Li, J., Zhang, B., Jia, W., Yang, M., Zhang, Y., Zhang, J., ... & Liu, W. (2021). Activation of adenosine monophosphate-activated protein kinase

drives the aerobic glycolysis in hippocampus for delaying cognitive decline following electroacupuncture treatment in APP/PS1 mice. *Frontiers in Cellular Neuroscience, 15*, 774569.

16. Huang, Q., Chen, R., Peng, M., Li, L., Li, T., Liang, F. X., & Xu, F. (2020). Effect of electroacupuncture on SIRT1/NF-κB signaling pathway in adipose tissue of obese rats. *Zhongguo Zhen jiu= Chinese Acupuncture & Moxibustion, 40*(2), 185-191.

17. Xu, J., Chen, L., Tang, L., Chang, L., Liu, S., Tan, J., ... & Cui, J. (2015). Electroacupuncture inhibits weight gain in diet-induced obese rats by activating hypothalamicLKB1-AMPK signaling. *BMC Complementary and Alternative Medicine, 15*, 1-9.

18. Tian, T., Sun, Y., Wu, H., Pei, J., Zhang, J., Zhang, Y., ... & Fan, C. (2016). Acupuncture promotes mTOR-independent autophagic clearance of aggregation-prone proteins in mouse brain. *Scientific Reports, 6*(1), 19714.

19. Zhang, H., Qin, F., Liu, A., Sun, Q., Wang, Q., Xie, S., ... & Lu, Z. (2019). Electro-acupuncture attenuates the mice premature ovarian failure via mediating PI3K/AKT/mTOR pathway. *Life Sciences, 217*, 169-175.

20. Kusuma, A. C., Oktari, N., Mihardja, H., Srilestari, A., Simadibrata, C. L., Hestiantoro, A., ... & Muna, N. (2019). Electroacupuncture enhances number of mature oocytes and fertility rates for in vitro fertilization. *Medical Acupuncture, 31*(5), 289-297.

21. Liu, P., Zhao, H., & Luo, Y. (2017). Anti-aging implications of Astragalus membranaceus (Huangqi): a well-known Chinese tonic. *Aging and disease, 8*(6), 868.

22. de Jesus, B. B., Schneeberger, K., Vera, E., Tejera, A., Harley, C. B., & Blasco, M. A. (2011). The telomerase activator TA-65 elongates short telomeres and increases health span of adult/old mice without increasing cancer incidence. *Aging cell, 10*(4), 604-621.

23. Zhang, X., Liang, T., Yang, W., Zhang, L., Wu, S., Yan, C., & Li, Q. (2020). Astragalus membranaceus injection suppresses production of interleukin-6 by activating autophagy through the AMPK-mTOR pathway in lipopolysaccharide-stimulated macrophages. *Oxidative Medicine and Cellular Longevity, 2020*.

5. Our Immune System: Defender and Slayer

1. Smith, B. (2018, May 21). Cold defense: getting inked may be the flashy new way to prevent the common cold. *Men's Journal*. https://www.mensjournal.com/health-fitness/how-getting-tattoos-weightlifting

2. Lynn, C. D., Dominguez, J. T., & DeCaro, J. A. (2016, March 4). Tattooing to "Toughen up": Tattoo experience and secretory immunoglobulin A. *American Journal of Human Biology, 28*(5), 599-602.

3. Richtel, M. (2019). *An elegant defense: the extraordinary new science of the immune system*. William Morrow. https://www.mattrichtel.com/an-elegant-defense

4. Velasquez-Manoff, M. (2012). *An epidemic of absence: A new way of understanding allergies and autoimmune diseases*. Simon and Shuster.

5. Richtel, M. (2019). *An elegant defense: the extraordinary new science of the immune system.* William Morrow. https://www.mattrichtel.com/an-elegant-defense

6. Abbas, A.K., Lichtman, A.H. & Pillai, S. (2015). *Cellular and molecular immunology.* Elsevier Saunders.

7. Richtel, M. (2019). *An elegant defense: the extraordinary new science of the immune system.* William Morrow. https://www.mattrichtel.com/an-elegant-defense

8. Abbas, A.K., Lichtman, A.H. & Pillai, S. (2015). *Cellular and molecular immunology.* Elsevier Saunders.

9. Richtel, M. (2019). *An elegant defense: the extraordinary new science of the immune system.* William Morrow. https://www.mattrichtel.com/an-elegant-defense

10. Velasquez-Manoff, M. (2012). *An epidemic of absence: A new way of understanding allergies and autoimmune diseases.* Scribner. https://books.google.mv/books?id=9eGxJe5OpOsC&printsec=frontcover&source=gbs_atb#v=onepage&q&f=false

11. Smallwood, T. B., Giacomin, P. R., Loukas, A., Mulvenna, J. P., Clark, R. J., & Miles, J. J. (2017). Helminth immunomodulation in autoimmune disease. *Frontiers in immunology, 8,* 453.

12. S Ding, S. S., Hong, S. H., Wang, C., Guo, Y., Wang, Z. K., & Xu, Y. (2014). Acupuncture modulates the neuro-endocrine-immune network. *QJM: An International Journal of Medicine, 107*(5), 341-345.

13. Chen, L. L. (Ed.). (2013). Acupuncture in Modern Medicine. InTech. doi: 10.5772/46017

14. McDonald, J. L., Smith, P. K., Smith, C. A., Xue, C. C., Golianu, B., Cripps, A. W., & Mucosal Immunology Research Group. (2016). Effect of acupuncture on house dust mite specific IgE, substance P, and symptoms in persistent allergic rhinitis. *Annals of Allergy, Asthma & Immunology, 116*(6), 497-505.

15. Min, S., Kim, K. W., Jung, W. M., Lee, M. J., Kim, Y. K., Chae, Y., ... & Park, H. J. (2019). Acupuncture for histamine-induced itch: association with increased parasympathetic tone and connectivity of putamen-midcingulate cortex. *Frontiers in neuroscience, 13,* 215.

16. Sparrow, K. (2007). Analysis of heart rate variability in acupuncture practice: Can it improve outcomes?. *Medical Acupuncture, 19*(1), 37-42.

6. Inflammation: Silent, Pervasive and Deadly

1. Blanco-Melo, D., Nilsson-Payant, B. E., Liu, W. C., Uhl, S., Hoagland, D., Møller, R., ... & Albrecht, R. A. (2020). Imbalanced host response to SARS-CoV-2 drives development of COVID-19. *Cell, 181*(5), 1036-1045.

2. Somers, J. (2020, November 2). How the coronavirus hacks the immune system. *New Yorker.* https://www.newyorker.com/magazine/2020/11/09/how-the-coronavirus-hacks-the-immune-system

3. Williams, D. P., Koenig, J., Carnevali, L., Sgoifo, A., Jarczok, M. N., Sternberg, E. M., & Thayer, J. F. (2019). Heart rate variability and inflammation: a meta-analysis of human studies. *Brain, behavior, and immunity, 80,* 219-226.

Notes

4. Pavlov VA, Wang H, Czura CJ, Friedman SG, Tracey KJ. The cholinergic anti-inflammatory pathway: a missing link in neuroimmunomodulation. Mol Med. 2003 May-Aug;9(5-8):125-34.

5. Huang, C. L., Tsai, P. S., Wang, T. Y., Yan, L. P., Xu, H. Z., & Huang, C. J. (2007). Acupuncture stimulation of ST36 (Zusanli) attenuates acute renal but not hepatic injury in lipopolysaccharide-stimulated rats. *Anesthesia & Analgesia, 104*(3), 646-654.

6. Da Silva, M. D., Bobinski, F., Sato, K. L., Kolker, S. J., Sluka, K. A., & Santos, A. R. (2015). IL-10 cytokine released from M2 macrophages is crucial for analgesic and anti-inflammatory effects of acupuncture in a model of inflammatory muscle pain. *Molecular neurobiology, 51*, 19-31.

7. Böbel, T. S., Hackl, S. B., Langgartner, D., Jarczok, M. N., Rohleder, N., Rook, G. A., Lowry, C. A., Gündel, H., Waller, C., & Reber, S. O. (2018). Less immune activation following social stress in rural vs. urban participants raised with regular or no animal contact, respectively. *Proceedings of the National Academy of Sciences of the United States of America, 115*(20), 5259–5264. https://doi.org/10.1073/pnas.1719866115

8. Ulloa, L., Quiroz-Gonzalez, S., & Torres-Rosas, R. (2017). Nerve stimulation: immunomodulation and control of inflammation. *Trends in molecular medicine, 23*(12), 1103-1120.

9. Torres-Rosas, R., Yehia, G., Peña, G., Mishra, P., del Rocio Thompson-Bonilla, M., Moreno-Eutimio, M. A., ... & Ulloa, L. (2014). Dopamine mediates vagal modulation of the immune system by electroacupuncture. *Nature medicine, 20*(3), 291-295.

10. Yang, N. N., Yang, J. W., Ye, Y., Huang, J., Wang, L., Wang, Y., ... & Liu, C. Z. (2021). Electroacupuncture ameliorates intestinal inflammation by activating α7nAChR-mediated JAK2/STAT3 signaling pathway in postoperative ileus. *Theranostics, 11*(9), 4078.

11. Zhang, L., Wu, Z., Zhou, J., Lu, S., Wang, C., Xia, Y., ... & Li, W. (2021). Electroacupuncture Ameliorates Acute Pancreatitis: A Role for the Vagus Nerve–Mediated Cholinergic Anti-Inflammatory Pathway. *Frontiers in Molecular Biosciences, 8*, 647647.

12. Liu, S., Wang, Z., Su, Y. *et al.* (2021) A neuroanatomical basis for electroacupuncture to drive the vagal–adrenal axis. *Nature*, 598, 641–645. https://doi.org/10.1038/s41586-021-04001-4

13. Williams, D. P., Koenig, J., Carnevali, L., Sgoifo, A., Jarczok, M. N., Sternberg, E. M., & Thayer, J. F. (2019). Heart rate variability and inflammation: a meta-analysis of human studies. *Brain, behavior, and immunity, 80*, 219-226.

14. Koopman, F. A., Tang, M. W., Vermeij, J., De Hair, M. J., Choi, I. Y., Vervoordeldonk, M. J., ... & Tak, P. P. (2016). Autonomic dysfunction precedes development of rheumatoid arthritis: a prospective cohort study. *EBioMedicine, 6*, 231-237.

15. Sajadieh, A., Nielsen, O. W., Rasmussen, V., Hein, H. O., Abedini, S., & Hansen, J. F. (2004). Increased heart rate and reduced heart-rate variability are associated with subclinical inflammation in middle-aged and elderly subjects with no apparent heart disease. *European heart journal, 25*(5), 363-370.

16. Adlan, A. M., van Zanten, J. J. V., Lip, G. Y., Paton, J. F., Kitas, G. D., & Fisher, J. P. (2017). Cardiovascular autonomic regulation, inflammation and pain in rheumatoid arthritis. *Autonomic Neuroscience, 208*, 137-145.
17. Sloan, R. P., McCreath, H., Tracey, K. J., Sidney, S., Liu, K., & Seeman, T. (2007). RR interval variability is inversely related to inflammatory markers: the CARDIA study. *Molecular medicine, 13*(3), 178-184.
18. Malave, H. A., Taylor, A. A., Nattama, J., Deswal, A., & Mann, D. L. (2003). Circulating levels of tumor necrosis factor correlate with indexes of depressed heart rate variability: a study in patients with mild-to-moderate heart failure. *Chest, 123*(3), 716-724.

7. When Pain Strikes

1. Simon, L. S. (2012). Relieving pain in America: a blueprint for transforming prevention, care, education, and research. *Journal of pain & palliative care pharmacotherapy, 26*(2), 197-198.
2. Centers for Disease Control and Prevention. (2022, May 11). *US overdose deaths in 2021 increased half as much as in 2020—but are still up 15%.* [Press release]. https://www.cdc.gov/nchs/pressroom/nchs_press_releases/2022/202205.htm
3. Hoffman, J. (2022, February 18). Sacklers raise their offer to settle opioid lawsuits by more than $1 billion. *New York Times.* https://www.nytimes.com/2022/02/18/health/sacklers-opioids-lawsuit.html?searchResultPosition=2
4. Shmerling, R.H. (2020, April 17). A new look at steroid injections for knee and hip osteoarthritis. *Harvard Health Blog.*
5. Kolata, G. (2019, May 15). How Tiger Woods won the back surgery lottery. *New York Times.* https://www.nytimes.com/2019/05/15/sports/how-tiger-woods-pga-back-surgery.html?searchResultPosition=1
6. How to Germany. (2022, Oct. 6). Spa: saunas per aquam an old roman cure. *Howtogermany.com.* https://www.howtogermany.com/pages/spas.html
7. Kolata, G. (2019, May 15). How Tiger Woods won the back surgery lottery. *New York Times.* https://www.nytimes.com/2019/05/15/sports/how-tiger-woods-pga-back-surgery.html?searchResultPosition=1
8. Suwen, N. (1995). *The Yellow Emperor's Classic of Medicine* (M. Ni PhD, Trans.). Shambala.
9. Neighmond, P. & Knox, R. (2014, January 13). *Pain in the back? Exercise may help you learn not to feel it* [Radio broadcast]. NPR. Pain In the Back? Exercise May Help You Learn Not To Feel It : Shots - Health News : NPR
10. Ibid.
11. Melzack R, Wall PD. Acupuncture and transcutaneous electrical nerve stimulation. Postgrad Med J. 1984 Dec;60(710):893-6.
12. Katz J, Rosenbloom BN. The golden anniversary of Melzack and Wall's gate control theory of pain: Celebrating 50 years of pain research and management. Pain Res Manag. 2015 Nov-Dec;20(6):285-6. doi: 10.1155/2015/865487. PMID: 26642069; PMCID: PMC4676495.

13. Li, Y., Yu, Y., Liu, Y., & Yao, W. (2022). Mast cells and acupuncture analgesia. *Cells*, *11*(5), 860.
14. In, S. L., Gwak, Y. S., Kim, H. R., Razzaq, A., Lee, K. S., Kim, H. Y., ... & Yang, C. H. (2016). Hierarchical micro/nano-porous acupuncture needles offering enhanced therapeutic properties. *Scientific Reports*, *6*(1), 34061.
15. Ciesielczyk, K., Furgała, A., Dobrek, Ł., Juszczak, K., & Thor, P. (2017). Altered sympathovagal balance and pain hypersensitivity in TNBS-induced colitis. *Archives of Medical Science*, *13*(1), 246-255.
16. https://ksparrowmd.com/shape-magazine-why-you-should-try-acupuncture-even-if-you-dont-need-pain-relief/
17. Mechling, L. (2021, June 28). Trying acupuncture for the first time helped pull me out of my quarantine fog. *Shape*. https://www.shape.com/lifestyle/mind-and-body/acupuncture-review-quarantine-fog
18. Harriott, A. M., & Schwedt, T. J. (2014). Migraine is associated with altered processing of sensory stimuli. *Current pain and headache reports*, *18*, 1-7.

8. Mood Disorders: Dissolving the Mind/Body Barrier

1. World Health Organization. (2021, June 17). One in 100 deaths is by suicide. https://www.who.int/news/item/17-06-2021-one-in-100-deaths-is-by-suicide
2. Witters, D., Liu, D. and Agrawal, S.. "Depression Costs U.S. Workplaces $23 Billion in Absenteeism." *Gallup*. July 24, 2013. https://news.gallup.com/poll/163619/depression-costs-workplaces-billion-absenteeism.aspx/
3. Hillhouse, T. M., & Porter, J. H. (2015). A brief history of the development of antidepressant drugs: from monoamines to glutamate. *Experimental and clinical psychopharmacology*, *23*(1), 1–21. https://doi.org/10.1037/a0038550
4. Moncrieff, J., Cooper, R.E., Stockmann, T., et al. *The serotonin theory of depression: a systematic umbrella review of the evidence. Mol Psychiatry (2022).*
5. Gafoor, R., Booth, H. P., & Gulliford, M. C. (2018). Antidepressant utilisation and incidence of weight gain during 10 years' follow-up: population based cohort study. *Bmj*, *361*.
6. Weight Gain and Antidepressants (Including SSRIs) (webmd.com)
7. Gao SY, Wu QJ, Zhang TN, Shen ZQ, Liu CX, Xu X, Ji C, Zhao YH. Fluoxetine and congenital malformations: a systematic review and meta-analysis of cohort studies. Br J Clin Pharmacol. 2017 Oct;83(10):2134-2147. https://www.drugwatch.com/ssri/birth-defects/ (2023).
8. Kwon, D. (2016, February 3). The hidden harm of antidepressants. *Scientific American.*
9. Sharma, T., Guski, L. S., Freund, N., & Gøtzsche, P. C. (2016). Suicidality and aggression during antidepressant treatment: systematic review and meta-analyses based on clinical study reports. *bmj*, *352*.
10. Ebrahim, S., Bance, S., Athale, A., Malachowski, C., & Ioannidis, J. P. (2016). Meta-analyses with industry involvement are massively published

and report no caveats for antidepressants. *Journal of clinical epidemiology*, *70*, 155-163.

11. Kwon, D. (2016, February 3). The hidden harm of antidepressants. *Scientific American*.

12. Yoo, S. D., & Park, E. J. (2022). Association of depressive and somatic symptoms with heart rate variability in patients with traumatic brain injury. *Journal of clinical medicine*, *12*(1), 104.

13. Liu, C. H., Zhang, G. Z., Li, B., Li, M., Woelfer, M., Walter, M., & Wang, L. (2019). Role of inflammation in depression relapse. *Journal of neuroinflammation*, *16*, 1-11.

14. Liu CH, Zhang GZ, Li B, Li M, Woelfer M, Walter M, Wang L. Role of inflammation in depression relapse. J Neuroinflammation. 2019 Apr 17;16(1):90. doi: 10.1186/s12974-019-1475-7. PMID: 30995920; PMCID: PMC6472093.

15. Tracey, K. & Bouton, C. (2022, June 6). From inflammation to depression, electricity is transforming medicine. *National Geographic*. https://www.nationalgeographic.com/magazine/article/from-inflammation-to-depression-electricity-is-transforming-medicine

16. Zamani M, Alizadeh-Tabari S, Zamani V. Systematic review with meta-analysis: the prevalence of anxiety and depression in patients with irritable bowel syndrome. Aliment. Pharmacol. Ther. 2019;50:132–143.

17. Oświęcimska J., Szymlak A., Roczniak W., Girczys-Połedniok K., Kwiecień J. New insights into the pathogenesis and treatment of irritable bowel syndrome. Adv. Med. Sci. 2017;62:17–30.

18. Bullmore, E. (2020, January 19). From depression to dementia, inflammation is medicine's new frontier. *The Guardian*. Retrieved 8/23/2023, from https://www.theguardian.com/commentisfree/2020/jan/19/inflammation-depression-mind-body

19. Dieleman GC, Huizink AC, Tulen JH, Utens EM, Tiemeier H. Stress reactivity predicts symptom improvement in children with anxiety disorders. J Affect Disord. 2016 May 15;196:190-9. doi: 10.1016/j.jad.2016.02.022. Epub 2016 Feb 9. PMID: 26926658.

20. Fantini-Hauwel, C., Batselé, E., Gois, C., & Noel, X. (2020). Emotion regulation difficulties are not always associated with negative outcomes on women: the buffer effect of HRV. *Frontiers in psychology*, *11*, 697.

21. Sun, H., Zhao, H., Ma, C., Bao, F., Zhang, J., Wang, D. H., ... & He, W. (2013). Effects of electroacupuncture on depression and the production of glial cell line–derived neurotrophic factor compared with fluoxetine: a randomized controlled pilot study. *The Journal of Alternative and Complementary Medicine*, *19*(9), 733-739.

22. Fiol-Veny, A., De La Torre-Luque, A., Balle, M., & Bornas, X. (2018). Altered heart rate regulation in adolescent girls and the vulnerability for internalizing disorders. *Frontiers in physiology*, *9*, 852.

9. Shooting for the Moon: Long Life, Great Health and New Strategies to Achieve Them

1. Trinh D-TT, Le H-LT, Bui M-MP, Thai K-M (2023) *Heart rate variability during auricular acupressure at the left sympathetic point on healthy volunteers: a pilot study.* *Front. Neurosci.* 17:1116154. doi:10.3389/fnins.2023.1116154.

10. Stoking the Flywheel: Small Steps, Big Results and the Power Law of Systems Synergy

1. Clear, J. (2019). *Atomic Habits: An Easy & Proven Way to Build Good Habits & Break Bad Ones.* Unabridged. [New York], Penguin Random House.
2. Swart, T. (2019, February 8). 3 simple habits that can protect your brain from cognitive decline. *Fast Company.* https://www.fastcompany.com/90303904/3-tips-to-slowing-down-cognitive-decline
3. Khera, A. V., Emdin, C. A., Drake, I., Natarajan, P., Bick, A. G., Cook, N. R., ... & Kathiresan, S. (2016). Genetic risk, adherence to a healthy lifestyle, and coronary disease. *New England Journal of Medicine, 375*(24), 2349-2358.
4. Khera, A. V., Emdin, C. A., Drake, I., Natarajan, P., Bick, A. G., Cook, N. R., ... & Kathiresan, S. (2016). Genetic risk, adherence to a healthy lifestyle, and coronary disease. *New England Journal of Medicine, 375*(24), 2349-2358.
5. Shimojo, G., Joseph, B., Shah, R., Consolim-Colombo, F. M., De Angelis, K., & Ulloa, L. (2019). Exercise activates vagal induction of dopamine and attenuates systemic inflammation. *Brain, behavior, and immunity, 75*, 181-191.
6. Laukkanen, J. A., Laukkanen, T., & Kunutsor, S. K. (2018). Cardiovascular and Other Health Benefits of Sauna Bathing: A Review of the Evidence. *Mayo Clinic proceedings, 93*(8), 1111-1121. https://doi.org/10.1016/j.mayocp.2018.04.008
7. Sinclair, D. & LaPlante, M.D. (2019). *Lifespan: why we age—and why we don't have to.* Atria Books. Page 107.
8. May, F. J., Baer, L. A., Lehnig, A. C., So, K., Chen, E. Y., Gao, F., ... & Stanford, K. I. (2017). Lipidomic adaptations in white and brown adipose tissue in response to exercise demonstrate molecular species-specific remodeling. *Cell reports, 18*(6), 1558-1572.
9. van Marken Lichtenbelt, W. (2017). Who is the Iceman? *Temperature, 4*(3), 202-205.
10. Sinclair, D. & LaPlante, M.D. (2019). *Lifespan: why we age—and why we don't have to.* Atria Books.
11. Swart, T. (2019, February 8). 3 simple habits that can protect your brain from cognitive decline. *Fast Company.* https://www.fastcompany.com/90303904/3-tips-to-slowing-down-cognitive-decline

Notes

12. Institute of Medicine (US) and National Research Council (US) Committee on the Framework for Evaluating the Safety of Dietary Supplements. *Dietary Supplements: A Framework for Evaluating Safety.* Washington (DC): National Academies Press (US); 2005. 1, Introduction and Background. https://www.ncbi.nlm.nih.gov/books/NBK216048/

13. Sparrow, K. (2019, August 7). 7 Supplements to Live Longer, Rejuvenate Cells, Stay Limber, and Avoid Illness. *Kristen Sparrow, MD Blog.* https://ksparrowmd.com/7-supplements-to-live-longer-rejuvenate-cells-stay-limber-and-avoid-illnesssupplements-updated-list/

14. Cox, P. A., & Metcalf, J. S. (2017). Traditional food items in Ogimi, Okinawa: L-serine content and the potential for neuroprotection. *Current nutrition reports, 6*, 24-31.

15. Healthnews Team. (2023, June 14). What are health influencers saying about the B-NMN supplement ban? *Healthnews.com.* https://healthnews.com/longevity/longevity-supplements/what-are-health-influencers-saying-about-the-b-nmn-supplement-ban/

16. de Jesus, B. B., Schneeberger, K., Vera, E., Tejera, A., Harley, C. B., & Blasco, M. A. (2011). The telomerase activator TA-65 elongates short telomeres and increases health span of adult/old mice without increasing cancer incidence. *Aging cell, 10*(4), 604-621.

17. FoundMyFitness Clips. *Bruce Ames on the importance of maintaining optimal vitamin D levels.* [Video]. YouTube. https://www.youtube.com/watch?v=NMx0CCDjukM

18. Mann, M. C., Exner, D. V., Hemmelgarn, B. R., Sola, D. Y., Turin, T. C., Ellis, L., & Ahmed, S. B. (2013). Vitamin D levels are associated with cardiac autonomic activity in healthy humans. *Nutrients, 5*(6), 2114-2127.

19. Walker, M. (2018). *Why we sleep: unlocking the power of sleep and dreams.* Scribner. https://www.simonandschuster.com/books/Why-We-Sleep/Matthew-Walker/9781501144325

20. Huberman Lab. (2021, September 19). *Toolkit for sleep.* Retrieved May 6, 2023, from https://hubermanlab.com/toolkit-for-sleep/

21. Pollan, M. (2021, July 6). The invisible addiction: is it time to give up caffeine? *The Guardian.* https://www.theguardian.com/food/2021/jul/06/caffeine-coffee-tea-invisible-addiction-is-it-time-to-give-up

22. Dr. Weil. *Breathing exercises: 4-7-8 breath.* [Video.] Retrieved May 6, 2023, https://www.drweil.com/videos-features/videos/breathing-exercises-4-7-8-breath/

23. Cell Reports Medicine| Volume 4, ISSUE 1, 100895, January 17, 2023, https://www.cell.com/cell-reports-medicine/pdfExtended/S2666-3791(22)00474-8

24. Wim Hof Method. *Wim Hof breathing exercises.* Retrieved May 23, 2023, https://www.wimhofmethod.com/breathing-exercises

Acknowledgments

I would like to thank my patients, whose lively interest and hearty support has helped immeasurably to complete this book. They are a ballast in my life and a source of inspiration, stories, friendship and deeper meaning.

There are more authors than I can possibly acknowledge whose work has helped and guided me. Matt Richtel for his beautiful book, *An Elegant Defense*, on Immunology which encouraged me to write about science for a lay audience. Stephen Pressfield for his invaluable book, *The War of Art* on dealing with the resistance that comes with creative undertakings. Moises Velasquez-Manoff for his bravery in life and his unique voice and story in *An Epidemic of Absence*. Many thanks to Rita Redberg, physician cardiologist, Oncologist Vinay Prasad, and journalist David Epstein who unflinchingly tell the truth about what the medical science actually says.

I need to thank my spectacular children so full of life, smarts and enthusiasms who make my life worth living. And particular thanks to my son who offered encouragement and perspective on the creative process from his own deep experience. And finally, thanks to my lovely, indomitable, relentlessly positive husband Kevin, the greatest living American.

About the Author

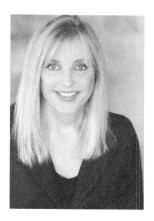

K. Sparrow, MD, is an author and board-certified pediatrician and anesthesiologist who now is a practicing acupuncturist. After getting a BA in biochemistry from UC Berkeley and working in a biochemistry lab on campus, she received her MD from Tulane University, completed her pediatrics residency at UCLA and her anesthesiology residency at UC Irvine. Sparrow was on staff and a partner at Kaiser San Francisco for more than a decade before a serious allergy caused her to change her careers. Today, Dr. Sparrow runs her own acupuncture practice in San Francisco, California. *Radical Resilience* is her first book.

Made in the USA
Las Vegas, NV
30 September 2024